Oral STD

Amanda Jones

DEDICATION

This book is dedicated to all those who are struggling with herpes. A cure is close and we hope to make it even closer by publishing this book. Proceeds from this book will fund Dr. Bryan Cullen of Duke University's research. We feel he is closest to finding a cure. We are willing to donate to other legitimate research facilities; please visit www.oralstd.webs.com for more information.

Note: To protect the innocent and not so innocent the names in this story have been changed.

.

ACKNOWLEDGMENTS

Thank you for all the love, support, and encouragement from family, and friends. This book would not be possible without you. Whether you know it or not, you have contributed to this book. The awareness ribbon find was especially greatly appreciated. Because of you, we can finally focus on finding a cure.

Chapter 1

Ahhh poker night. A time for me to unwind and truly be me. There will be cigar smoking, swearing, drinking, crude jokes, your typical den of iniquity when the guys get together. The only thing – I am not a guy. I am a woman. A mother of two teenagers, Sandra and David. Growing up the youngest of 5 males, gave me the comfortably among men that many women do not have. At poker night, I truly am "one of the guys." There will be the occasional "why do women" questions which is fine because it allows me to ask my "why do men" questions. Growing up around my brothers, I do know a lot about men, and am a pretty good lie detector when it comes to them. However, I have grown to be grateful for my poker nights as I can ask specific questions that my brothers never would answer – on the count of still being considered the "baby sister."

How did I arrive here? My life started off the perfect fairy tale. I married my high school sweet heart, Charles Jones, right after high school graduation. He worked two jobs so I could go back to school to obtain my dream job as a technical writer. He then continued to work the two jobs, until we had saved enough for a down-payment on a house. My technical writer position allowed me to work from home, giving me time for the children we planned on having, as well as be a "traditional housewife." Although I grew up being a tomboy, I am very old-fashioned and have no problem doing the cooking and housework. However, my husband felt he should at least participate in some of the household chores, and I'd often find certain tasks done before I could start them. I was truly spoiled. My friends, used to tease me to clone my husband, as there are "not many like him."

My life was truly a dream, until I was forced to "wake up" by the drunk driver who took Charlie from me. That was probably the first devastating life event for me. The second you will see at the end of my story.

Eventually, I started dating again. I didn't think I could do it, but I received encouragement from my family, friends, and even my in-laws. What many people do not realize is when children are in the picture, you really are not dating for yourself, but your children as well. I have to be more selective when I date. I have a strict policy that I will not introduce anyone to my kids unless I know the guy is in it for the "long haul." I do not want my children exposed to a revolving door of men.

I have several friends who set me up on the occasional blind date with a "great guy," but there was always something that never really clicked. Then there would be the guy who I would date for months, and he would pressure me to meet my kids. I would ask if he saw the relationship really going somewhere, at which point he would drop the subject, then drop me. That mystery I could never quite solve.

What has made my dating life easier are my two single best friends, Julie and Rob who are still "in the trenches" with me. Julie and I have been friends since 1st grade. She coming from, at that time, the only African American family in the neighborhood, and me being a tomboy were natural outcasts. You will never meet a more highly educated woman, who is down-to-earth and approachable. She has a top-secret job working as a consultant for the government.

One of those, I could tell you what I do, but then I would have to kill you. A perfect job fit as she is thorough, intelligent, and generous, but cross her or a loved one – a Tasmanian devil will attack you.

Rob was the only openly gay male at the time in our high school. An outcast as well, his athletic talents gave him access to areas many homosexual students at the time would not have. His only supportive family member is his mother. Julie and I filled the void left by his siblings and father. He is a high powered sports attorney. He claims he uses all the homophobic hatred that has been hurled at him, and uses it to propel himself forward in his career. Cross him, or someone he loves, and you will live to regret it. We are thick as thieves, and stand by each other, no matter the situation.

My parents, brothers and in-laws have all moved. Mostly to warm states: Louisiana, Florida, Arizona and California. They've tried to get me to relocate, but I do not fare well in the heat. We all keep in touch via Facebook, email, Skype, Oovoo, you name it, and we've done it. To make sure our children remain close, for two weeks in the summer, someone will host all of "the kids." My parents usually go to whichever location as well to help. I just did my two weeks last year. This year my kids are going to Arizona.

I am also lucky enough to have the most caring, and personable in-laws ever. After my husband's death and when they still lived nearby, I would often attend family functions with them. My mother-in-law would point out several men who were "checking me out." I would always wrinkle my face and say "Mom, he's with his girlfriend." She would roll her eyes and say "oh honey, please! He's not married yet." It took her telling me this several times, for me to take notice. Several of the women one and two generations ahead of me had the same slogan. A slogan that has evolved into what my friends and I have termed "serial dating."

I laughed at this "eureka" moment with Julie and Rob. I never noticed this growing up with my brothers, but as we reflected on it one evening, there were constantly girlfriends in and out of the house. Even when there was a "serious girlfriend" there was always another girlfriend on "the side." I never gave my brothers up as I love them fiercely, and well the girlfriends were all obeying my every whim, so I was in heaven. I was constantly receiving gifts and I somehow knew early not to overturn the gravy boat.

Julie, Rob and I decided to adopt this strategy – we figured it was to be much easier to serial date, especially when time is limited. Rob even stated that this was the way in the gay lifestyle. You can weed out the bad ones, but still have some "that you are working on." Rob was, at one point, dating 4 guys at the same time. Unfortunately, they did not amount to much and he weeded them all out, but that's for another story. We label the ones we are dating as "potentials" and we do not use their names until they get pass the weeding out process. We even give them nicknames. As Rob says, why bother remembering names, if they are going to be gone in a few months?

Do not get me wrong, we are looking for a healthy, committed relationship. But who has time to date someone for years on end, only to have it not amount to anything? With serial dating, you can better weigh your options. Trust ME ladies, guys do it all the time. You might be lucky enough to be with the 1 percent of the male population that is faithful and committed since day one, but ladies– "don't waste your pretty." Another slogan I learned from the female generations ahead of me. Do not get bogged down to one person, until they are ready to fully commit to you – with a marriage proposal. Unfortunately marriage will not make a man commit to you 100% either, but at least you have some legal recourse if that relationship doesn't work. Julie, Rob and I are honest with our potentials about dating other people. Rob is a huge believer in karma. Note: Serial dating does not mean serial sexual relationships. Serial dating is simply not putting all your eggs in one basket.

If you also happen to just be out of a relationship, and not really looking right now, serial dating is the best way to get back on your feet. It allows you to test the waters, and in my case, get people off your back about you "moving on." When I first started serial dating, I was at a point in my life where I was not looking for a sexual relationship; but I have to admit, I was missing adult male company. No offense to Rob, as he gives good hugs, however, I was actually missing the romantic aspects of being in a relationship.

Chapter 2

But I digress. I just felt it was essential to fill in some of the blanks. Back to poker night. A tradition for well over 10 years now. It was always hosted at one of, as we called ourselves, "the fab 5's"home. The other four were made up of John, Alvin, Alex, and Ben. Others would come and go, but we would remain the same. They were my husband's closest friends. When my husband was alive, I was invited to join them at the games. I wouldn't attend every game as I felt it was important for my husband to have his "man time." After my husband passed, they insisted I continue to play. Everyone was responsible for bringing an alcoholic beverage and something to eat. I often wonder if they allowed me to stay because I always had actual food and not the chips and pretzels they usually bring.

The games were always entertaining and comfortable for me. That is until Michael showed up one evening. Michael was your tall, dark and handsome type. I did notice him right away, but I knew the guys warned new players that I was off-limits. So I respected their policy, and never flirted with the new guys, not that I wanted to flirt with the previous ones. There was however an instant physical attraction to Michael, the kind you feel in "your gut." This truly was the first newcomer that I checked out from head to toe. I had conflicting feelings. If the guys protected me from the "losers" that showed up, I should not be throwing myself at the first "hottie." Somehow it came out in the introduction that he was engaged. That quickly ended the attraction, engaged equals married to me. He is "hands-off" in the serial dating world.

Michael was quiet the first couple of games. I just attributed his silence to the usual uncomfortableness of having a woman during "man's night out," and not knowing what to say. John said he was a child psychologist and he met him at the school where he teachers. It usually doesn't take the new players long to fall in with the teasing and joking, so I wasn't too concerned.

Fast-forward several months after Michael's arrival, the joking started to change, probably after the third game. It seemed as if Michael was showing an interest in me. Michael really could not be flirting with me? I decided it was my imagination. The other guys usually nipped that in the bud, when a new guy slipped, and forgot the rules. Since the other guys didn't protest, I decided it was all in my head.

At the fourth game, it seemed as if the flirting became more obvious, and the guys were even encouraging the flirting. In fact, during one hand it came down to just Michael and me. Michael's pot was much bigger than mine. So I had to "go all in." I had three aces, so I was not backing down. Before I had a chance to push my money in the pot, John joked, "Amanda, why don't you just offer to kiss him instead, I'm sure he prefers that over the money."

I panicked and looked at Michael who quickly dropped his eyes to the cards in his hand, he seemed as if he was more embarrassed than me.

"You'd probably like to see that John, but we'd have to

charge you," was my response.

The rest of the guys laughed and Michael folded. I happened to win most of the hands that night, but I couldn't celebrate as I was a bit uncomfortable by John's statement. Michael is engaged. Right? Next month was my turn to host poker night. I will feel "safer" in my own space; perhaps I can turn the tables somehow and get the bottom of what was happening. I have a dinner with Julie and Rob, and a couple of my kid's basketball games to get me through the next couple of weeks. I can discuss this episode with Julie and Rob, get their feedback. I decide my best bet is to cash out and leave, tell them they need their "man time." Part of being considered "one of the guys" is knowing when you're really not and back out the room.

Chapter 3

I arrive home early. Early enough to find Sandra and David watching a movie in the family room.

"What are you doing home so early? Lady luck not with you?" David asks.

If only that was the reason, I think. "Actually, Mr. Smarty-pants, she was with me big time, I just know when not to push a good thing."

"We're about to have a Star Trek marathon if you want to join us. Oh, and Aunt Julie called she said don't forget about dinner tomorrow. It has been moved up to 4:00 because Uncle Rob has to fly out right after." Sandra interrupts.

"A Star Trek marathon sounds like exactly what I need. You two start and I'll join you after I've showered." I respond. I originally had planned on relaxing and emptying my thoughts during a hot bubble bath, but bonding with my kids over sci-fi was a far better option.

In the shower I go over the poker game comment from John in my head. I decide I've misread their teasing. That is all it is. Just teasing. No need to bring it up with Rob and Julie, it is just my mind playing tricks. Who wouldn't want an extremely attractive man to show an interest in them? I end my shower, then join my kids in the family room. We never make it to the Captain Picard movies and all fall asleep in the room. I eventually wake to the smell of bacon, cinnamon rolls and coffee in the morning. That could only mean one thing. Julie is here.

I open my eyes to see Sandra and David still asleep. I decide to leave them. The smell of Julie's cooking will wake them soon enough. Julie and I have been friends for so long, we're really like sisters. We have keys to each other's homes and think nothing of going right in and making ourselves comfortable. Luckily for my kids and me, Julie's idea of making herself comfortable is coming in and cooking a meal. Cooking is a stress reliever for her. She just hates cooking for one person. We never know when she's coming. We just know we're usually stuffed and satiated when she's gone.

"Morning Mandy." Julie beams. My childhood nickname. My kids often joke they know how long someone knows me, by what name they call me.

"I found this caramel cream sugar I wanted to try on some cinnamon rolls. What will it be for breakfast, I figured bacon and eggs? Nothing too fancy since I have the cinnamon rolls?"

Julie cooking is a sight to behold. A tall attractive woman with Sofia Vergara curves stands in my kitchen wearing an apron and immaculately dressed. There is never a wrinkle in her clothes, or a lock of her hair that is out of place. She is plugged in to her iPod as she feels music helps her create in the kitchen.

When she's in her full on cooking mode, there is really no stopping her - on extremely rare instances you are allowed to assist. Our deal has been, she does the cooking and we're responsible for the cleanup. Although the control freak in her cleans as she goes, so there is usually minimal to do.

"How about those red velvet waffles you made last time?"

I turn to see David has entered the kitchen. As usual, he is the first one at any meal.

"Anything for my favorite nephew." Julie responds.

"I'm your only nephew." David answers.

"That's why you're my favorite." Julie replies. "Red velvet waffles it is!"

Julie disappears to the pantry and comes out with a mixing bowl, flour, and various other ingredients. David grabs the plates and silverware and begins to set the table.

"Oh good! I was hoping you'd show up this morning Aunt Julie." Sandra has now entered, her eyes are still half closed. "I forgot to ask you something."

"Yes Sandy my love?"

Only four people are allowed to call her Sandy: Julie, John, David and Rob. She often questions why she was given a name that has a rhyme potential with mine. I remind her it was her father's grandmother's name, which never seems to satisfy her. I just attribute her constant questions to teenager angst.

Julie turns to look at Sandra. With Sandra up, she can now plug her iPod into the speakers she gave us one Christmas as a "house present." She has eclectic taste, so you never know what is going to be on her playlist. It can be anything from classical, to pop, to gangster rap. She claims you never know where you are going to find your inspiration, so take advantage of it all.

"Next month is Black History Month, and we have to write

about someone from history who we admire. I rather not do that, since my teacher stressed it has to be someone we admire I got permission from my teacher to write about you."

I could tell Julie was touched because for a nanosecond, she lost her composure. Someone who doesn't know her like I do would've never seen it. She turned to Sandra and held her arms out to grab Sandra in a bear hug. "Of course, it would be my pleasure. I'm so honored you asked me."

As we sit down to eat the feast Julie has prepared for us, the topic of conversation is about upcoming basketball games. Julie whips out her Blackberry and plugs in the information. "Hmmmmm, looks like I'll be able to make a lot of the games this season! Awesome! How are the classroom grades?"

"Like you didn't hack into the high school computer system already?" David snorts.

"David Jones! Would I do that?" Julie replies while blinking her eyelashes.

Truth be told she wouldn't. Unless she felt our lives were at stake. Her job gives her access to all sorts of information, and it appears she has a high security level. Often times she has asked me if I want to see their grades before the report card is printed, but luckily I don't have to worry about their grades. If they want to play sports, they have to be on honor roll. I am pretty sure Julie does a full background check on their teachers, but I can't quite prove it. Although she never discusses the details of her job, we often tease her about it.

"Look at the time! I have to get my workout in. Who wants to join me at the gym?" Julie asks.

We all three groan in unison. The last thing you think about after one of Julie's meals is going to the gym.

"Going back to bed." My kids say.

"I have a project I want to finish before we go out tonight." I respond.

Julie chuckles. "So be it. Mandy I'll pick you up at 3:00. I told Rob we'd drop him off at the airport after dinner."

"Sounds good." I respond, not sure how I'm going to eat later I'm so stuffed.

I head to my home office to finish up a project. Time seems to fly by and at 1:30 I decide to jump in the shower to get ready for dinner. Julie is always on time, and since I was still stuffed from breakfast, I decide I want to take my time getting ready. At exactly 3:00 she pulls in my driveway. I yell to my kids that I was going out, and head out to her car.

We drive over to Rob's house singing disco music from the 70's. Rob lives in the trendy part of town, so we almost always eat dinner by his apartment. We decide on a local tapas place. I send him a text to let him know we are 5 minutes away, and by the time we pull up, he is out front speaking with his doorman. The doorman gives us a polite wave – we both have keys to Rob's apartment and know all the doormen in the building.

"How are my lovely ladies?" Rob asks while climbing in the back. "Julie, honey, I doubt you are going to find parking at this time, so let's put the car in a parking lot, my treat. I'm STARVED! There is a good one right around the corner from the restaurant." Julie wrinkles her face at him.

Both my best friends are control freaks. You never know when they are going to agree or disagree. When they do have their arguments, they are very minor, and always over quickly. It appears Julie is not going to argue with him tonight, and makes her way over to the restaurant.

The restaurant seems to be a bit crowded tonight, but Rob is well known. He has "graced the palm" of many a maître d' or waiter with a ticket to a sporting event, or a big tip. As a result, when we walk in we are ushered right to a table.

"So, let's get into it. I haven't seen my boos in a couple of days. Who has any hot potentials?" Rob begins.

I've already decided not to mention Michael. I'll let them do all the talking.

"I got nothing." Julie states after sipping on her sangria.

"Ditto." I chime in.

"I got something." Rob responds. "He's a bit nerdy. An economist. But I'm going to try a good guy for once and see what happens."

"Nerdy? How nerdy is he compared to a lawyer?" Julie teases.

"He's also a Republican." Rob starts. "Hello! A gay Republican spells issues."

"I'm sure there are gay Republicans that don't have any issues!" I protest. "Give him a chance, opposites do attract. He could be the one."

"I could do a profile on him?" Julie suggests.

"NO!" Rob answers. "Hellooooo, way too stalkerish! Boy! Am I glad I met you in high school, I'd have a complex that you got references before you became my friend. Oh before I forget, I'll be out of town for Valentines, won't be able to do the ménage."

"Even if you were in town, you might be tied up with a certain economist." I tease.

Rob rolls his eyes and sticks his tongue out at me. Our

Valentines ménage is a long tradition. We are not sure how or when it started. Basically, we have a sleepover party for whoever is not in a relationship at the time. The past 4 Valentines Days, we've been a threesome. We rotate homes. My kids are also invited. We stay up all night gorging on decadent food Julie and/or Rob have prepared and watching movies. This year it is at my house.

"Uh-oh! There's Eric at 4:00 pm. Oh no, he's is NOT walking this way!" Rob and I freeze, not really wanting to turn around and show interest. Eric was Rob's boyfriend of two years. He broke up with Rob because "he wasn't in love." That is after Rob purchased him a new car, and got him a job. We could see Julie giving him a look of death.

"That's right bitch walk the other way." Julie seems to give one last death stare. "He's no longer walking this way." She says.

"You are the only one that can get away with calling a man a bitch." Rob says to lighten the mood. Julie gives him an evil all-knowing smile. Disaster avoided. I'm sure Rob is over him, but it really seemed they were in it for the long haul. Those types of love die hard. We spend the rest of the dinner and the drive to the airport chatting about Rob's new potential.

Chapter 4

I wake the next day with a nervous feeling in my stomach. I'm hosting the next poker night, which is soon. What should I wear? What am I going to cook? I have two weeks to plan it. February being the shortest month, with the most vacation days because of school closings, we always have the poker game the first weekend.

When I host the games, I cook a full meal. The guys know this, so they usually just bring the beverages and disposable eating utensils. Because I am home, cooking, and comfortable, I am "plain Jane" and wear over-sized sweats. I found my "comfortable look" to be rather dowdy; however, I'm usually exhausted from all the cooking and playing and it makes jumping into bed A LOT easier. I don't even put my contacts in, I wear my glasses. The look will probably send Michael packing. Maybe I should wear something else? Ugh! WAIT! He's engaged! How could I have forgotten that part? Someone did mention it at the first introduction. Okay, I'm relieved. More proof that the flirting was all in my head! Plain Jane look stays!

I pull out my Blackberry to figure out when I can go grocery shopping and prepare the meal in between my kids' basketball games. So I have 4 games, and a play audition. Not too bad.

The two weeks fly by with David's team winning one and losing one. Sandra's team won both games. Plus there was the practice for Sandra's auditions. Poker night finally arrives.

Sandra and David decide to go to Julie's house for the night. Sandra, to finish her project for Black History month. David, because Julie always has the latest electronic devices and allows him to "play" with them. I have a full spread laid out, appetizers, salad, and chicken cordon bleu. I even bake a cake. Now I just need my poker partners. John is the first to arrive. One by one the other guys arrive and it is business as usual. I am in the zone, and my mojo has returned. That is, until Michael enters.

"You look really hot" was the reaction I received when he walked through the door. All that money spent on my "sexy" clothes to think all I had to do was throw on sweats and pull my hair back in a bun to attract the attention of a "hottie?" I need to send a letter to the editor of Cosmopolitan STAT. Oh! Of course! He has to be joking. I'm sure to "hear it" from the other guys. So I wait for what seems like an awkward eternity. No one comments. So to break the awkwardness, or at least the awkwardness that I was feeling, I say the first thing that comes to mind.

"Ah, thanks Michael. So your fiancée is this smart librarian, or scientist type?"

"I'm not engaged, and actually she's pretty dumb." He replies.

Hmm, that was totally not the answer I was expecting. There was something there bugging me, perhaps the "dumb" comment? Guys do complain freely to each other about women they are dating, but they would never say anything so negative. This has become very confusing. I'm going to have to ask John. We're due to go grocery shopping soon. In fact, the Monday after next, as I quickly take a peek at my Blackberry. John is probably planning a romantic dinner for someone for Valentine's Day. So all I have to do is get through the night, and corner John later. I can do this. I'm not intimidated. After all, I have two teenagers.

Everyone grabs a plate to eat, and then we sit down at the table to begin playing.

"You all just need to hand over your wallets now. Lady Luck is with me tonight." Ben announces through a mouth full of food.

"Yeah, how much did YOU pay her?" Alex responds.

Insults continue to be traded back and forth across the table. The topic of conversation soon switches to what type of flowers a guy should get for Valentine's Day to get bonus points. I told them that it depends on the individual. It also depends on the type of relationship. Some women will read a lot into red roses. I could care less about them. My favorites are calla lilies, irises, and gerbera daisies. I know, a rather odd combination, but it is me. There was no "flirting" from Michael, so I relaxed. He didn't really seem to glance at me much during the game. I'm getting so many mixed signals from him. I will make John spill the beans when we're shopping.

The rest of the evening goes by with no sign of interest from Michael, and Ben actually being the big winner. Alex lost all his money half-way through, so the guys made him stay behind to help me clean up. Cleaning was done rather quickly since all we did was pick up the ends of the disposable table cloth and throw everything in it away. Alex thanked me for the evening and headed out the door. I threw myself in bed and fell asleep immediately.

Chapter 5

Two basketball games with Julie, a second audition for Sandra, and a martial arts belt ceremony for David and Sandra later, I meet John for our grocery shopping trip. If it were not for our trips, John would be surviving off of beer and potato chips. Our grocery shopping trips began when he read an article that women love a man that can cook. He also realized it was a lot cheaper than going to a restaurant. He was really green in the beginning. I would have to suggest foods to buy, and give him recipes. He has actually come a long way. He even watches the cooking network, and uses actual cooking terms.

"Ok dude! What is the deal with Michael and his relationship?" I ask once we are out of the car. John is a very aggressive driver, so I don't do too much speaking in the car, as he is usually yelling out the window.

"Oh please!" He replies. "That is such a bootleg relationship. He has been with her for 7 years and has never met her parents, family, or friends? Maureen is scared to introduce him because they are different religions. She mentioned him once, and they flipped out and threatened to disown her."

Ah, well I guess her name is Maureen. I'm not too comfortable knowing her name.

"Really? Because of religious differences? How different are the religions?" I ask.

"Let's not pretend like major wars have not been started over different religious views." John answers. "As different as polytheism and monotheism."

"So why doesn't he just break up with her?" I ask.

"I think he has some guilt complex about taking her virginity. But he is totally bored. Don't take this the wrong way, eh, I can totally tell you. You are not the first he has dated while with her. There are a good 5 before you, or at least 5 that I know of. But those chicks were flakey. He was even busted once out with one of them, but he totally made up some story about her being a colleague, and Maureen believed it."

"John, I am not buying that 100 percent. If he is so miserable, then why not break up with her? Why lead her along? Especially if you are dating other people and you're bored?"

"He's a really nice guy, and I think someone like you could help him see how miserable he really is. Come on, he's been with her for seven years, and never met her parents? Just a sibling and one or two friends? And don't give me if they get married and have a baby, a kid will make it better crap. That only makes it worse."

Although I was uncomfortable with Michael calling Maureen stupid, all I could hear was "honey, he's not married yet." I haven't been on a date in a good couple of months. He could be a potential. What do I have to lose really? The guys seem to like him. I decide at that moment I would try one date, but let him make the first move. I did not want to be the aggressor. Wait, not even sure he's interested.

"NICE! PURPLE ASPARAGUS! Hey do you think they have frozen avocado halves here?" John's comments snap me out of my thoughts.

"And what are you going to do with those my friend?" I ask.

"I will sauté the asparagus in a nice garlic butter sauce, the avocado is for a salad – I just need half of one. Not sure if you are aware, but avocados turn brown once cut open. That's why the frozen avocado halves work." He teases.

"So, without sounding like a teenage girl, Michael is interested in me?" I ask.

"Hey can we go to Trader Joes for some mango sorbet, that stuff is so refreshing after a big meal!" John ignores me.

"Not until you answer my question." I respond.

"Fine!" John sighs. "Yes, he's interested. Can we go to TJ's now?"

"Yes we can go get your mango sorbet." I respond. "I think it was Trader Joes that had the frozen avocado halves anyway."

"Excellent! Let's pay."

We pay for our items, and John being the perfect gentleman, always insists I get in the car as he unloads the groceries. Which is fine with me as it gives me time to prepare for his driving. I throw on my dark sunglasses as he drives, so I can close my eyes. I have a silent mental debate with myself on whether I should ask him about Michael's "she's dumb" comment.

"So back to Michael." He says as we pull out of the parking lot. "Me and the guys feel he's a good guy, and you should go for it. You are a great person and have a lot to offer."

I always get nervous when he speaks to me while driving. I try to keep it short and sweet. "I'll think about it no…"

"Look at this idiot!" John interrupts while leaning on the horn, forcing me to open my eyes. "It's a stop sign NOT a light!" He yells.

"No promises." I finish. "Why did he call her dumb?" I ask. John really isn't about to run this red light is he? I glance in the side view mirror and see a camera flash. I decide to sit back in the chair and close my eyes again.

"Oh, totally no pressure, it is purely your decision. He said it because she is stupid. She believes every word he says. Also very boring, not much conversation there."

A few minutes later, we pull into the Trader Joes parking lot.

"Are you getting anything?" John asks.

"Yes, I'm going to pick up some snacks for the kids, and I think I'll get some of that sweet corn."

I don't really need anything, but I always like to a good body stretch after I get out of John's car. I've tried suggesting I drive, but he tells me he wants to do "the man thing."

We seem to have a silent agreement not to talk about Michael anymore, which is fine with me. I have a lot of thinking to do. I will still wait for him to make the first move. While in Trader Joes, John tells me about the four women he's currently dating. However he's hoping for a more serious relationship with the one who gets the Valentine's dinner.

"What are you going to tell the others?" I ask.

"Originally, I was going to tell them I have a conference out of town, but I'm hoping dinner goes well. If so, I'm getting rid of two of them. Those two will know the truth."

"You're telling them after Valentine's Day?"

"Well yeah, I'm going to come down with a cold." John answers while speaking through his nose.

"Wouldn't it be easier to be honest with them, and tell them you are dating other people?" I ask.

"Oh hell no!" John responds. "Tried that once. Honesty is not always the best policy."

I make a face and we both laugh. We finish shopping, pay for our groceries, and then John drops me off home.

"Good luck cooking, if you need help, I'll be home Valentine's Day." I tell him.

"Thanks Mandy. My love to the kids! Catch you later!" John replies as his tires screech out of my driveway.

Chapter 6

Blah! Valentine's Day. Or as I've come to call it "Single Awareness Day." I can't take full credit for that title. I actually saw it on a news broadcast. I wouldn't get out of bed, except Julie is coming over for our ménage. As I stretch to ponder what lazy time I'm going to greet the world, Sandra comes bounding in my room with an enormous floral arrangement of calla lilies, irises, and gerbera daisies. Not really the prettiest combination, but someone obviously knows what I like, and spent a lot of money to put a smile on my face. Of course! It has to be Sandra and David.

Before I could thank her, she waives a card in the air and asks "Who is Michael?"

"You read my card?" I respond shocked. Not so much by her reading my card, but by Michael sending me flowers, and all my favorites.

"No offense, I thought they were for me." She laughs. "Maybe you should give him a shot, really Mom, stop worrying about us. We want you to be happy. Any guy who went through this much trouble should get at least one date!"

"Thanks sweetie, but I'm not that far gone where I'm going to start taking dating advice from you. What are you plans for the day? Aunt Julie is coming over if you want to stay and watch movies with us."

"Thanks, but David and I have plans to go to dinner and movies with friends."

"Tell David he can take the car if he wants."

"Ok, thanks Mom!"

The flowers give me the energy to pull myself out of bed. I decide to put them in the dining room. I have to call Michael to thank him for the flowers, but not with my kids around. They have practice today, so I know I don't have to wait too long. Plus I need time to go over possible conversation scenarios in my head, so I don't sound too much like an idiot.

Once I know I'm alone in the house I find the courage to call Michael to thank him and wish him a Happy Valentine's Day. As the phone rings, Julie walks in with movies and ice cream. When we first started our ménage, Julie insisted we have "hottie" themes. Last year was Lord of the Rings. This year it is British men, we narrowed our list down to Idris Elba, Jason Statham, and Daniel Craig. Rob sent us a text that he would try to video conference us.

Michael answers the phone before I can hang up. I hadn't planned on speaking to him in front of Julie.

"Michael, uh hi! It is Amanda. I just wanted to thank you for the gorgeous flowers and wish you a happy Valentine's Day."

I could see Julie raising her eyebrows and making questioning faces at me. She figures out this is a new potential. She knows enough to leave the room, so I can have some privacy. Besides, it is not like I won't tell her what is going on anyway.

27

She and I have shared so much in life and for so long; we could have full conversations without saying a word. She leaves the room, and returns a few minutes later to see if I am still on the phone, holding the flowers. She points to the phone. I nod my head. The face she makes says "this is the ugliest arrangement I have even seen, but at least he got all your favorite flowers and looks like he spent a lot of money. Hurry up and get off the phone and spill the beans." She exits quickly.

"You're welcome. I hope you like them. A little bird told me they were your favorites."

I giggle. "Smart little bird." I respond. "They were a pleasant surprise."

"I'm glad you like them. I was hoping they would make you feel guilty so you'd go on a date with me." Michael states.

"You don't have to make me feel guilty. I will go willingly."

"How does this Friday sound?"

"Tomorrow?" I ask.

"Oh, sorry, is it too soon?" He replies.

"No, I just wanted to be sure. It is a date." I say. "Is it possible I can call you back tomorrow to confirm? My friend Julie is here."

"Sure, call me whenever you want." He responds.

My conversation with Michael seemed very easy and free flowing, I didn't need any of the scenarios I practiced. Was it perhaps because Michael and I have known each other for a while, and the barriers were down? I am not quite sure. But it felt very comfortable, almost too comfortable. Why was I worrying? I had

John's reassurance he was a great guy. Wait! He did say call whenever I wanted. Wouldn't that be a bit awkward? What if he was with Maureen? Before I could dwell on the subject too long, Julie returns.

"Soooooooooo who's Michael, and how did he know what flowers to get?" She asks, while reading the card.

"He's one of the guys from the poker game." I respond.

I pause as she hates that I go to the games because she had dated someone with a huge gambling problem. He hid it from her for 2 years, which is an almost impossible feat to do with her. But when in love, you tend to overlook the important details sometimes. This was before we started serial dating, and it helped validate the need to serial date.

"WAIT! The guys are cool with this? Who is this guy?" She asks. She knew they were protective of me.

"He's a counselor. He works with kids, mostly teenagers. The guys actually encouraged it." I answer.

"Hmph, well okay, you know how I feel about gambling, but I don't think the guys would allow anyone to talk to you if he was not a decent human being. Have you been out with this guy? What's the next step?"

"We have a date Friday, we just made it."

"Do you need me to pick up the kids?" She asks.

I laugh. She is a bit overprotective of them. "You know, they are old enough to be by themselves. But thanks for the offer."

"Not a problem sister. Soooo before we watch our hot British men movies, let's go raid that closet of yours and see what you have to wear. Actually, let me mix up some drinks first, and then we'll have a look."

After a good twenty minutes, we settle on an emerald green snug wrap shirt with black pants. Plus it is clean, so no trip to the cleaners. Bonus! I had a giddiness that I have not had since my teenage years. What am I getting myself into? One date couldn't hurt me right?

Rob video conferenced us, as I was changing back into my sweats. "Hi ladies! I can't stay long I met some hot new potential on the plane. I just wanted to wish my favorite ladies a Happy V-Day! What the hell?! Why is Mandy half naked? Did you two cross over without telling me?"

"Noooooooooooooooo." We say in unison. "I have a date. I was trying on outfits. You go entertain your hottie, I'll tell you about it when you return." I reply.

"He can wait." Rob snaps. "I want the details."

Before I could answer, Julie responds. "His name is Michael, he's a therapist or something or other, she met him at the poker game. I will do a full workup on him later."

"Ah! So he's prescreened! Very nice. So there's less of a chance he's a loser. I'm sure the guys would've squashed it if he was." Rob states.

"Unless he has them fooled, I'll find out." Julie replies.

Rob and I both laugh. "Really Julie, it is okay. Let's see where this goes before you do anything. We could go out, and I could be completely bored, annoyed, disgusted, etc. Rob you go enjoy yourself."

"You know I will!" He answers.

"Love ya!" All three of us say in unison, and Rob hangs up

the call. Julie and I spend the rest of the evening ogling Jason and Idris and giggling like teenagers. We unfortunately never make it to Daniel Craig. We pass out in the wee hours of the morning in my bedroom.

Chapter 7

The next morning I wake to the smell of bacon. Julie is up with my kids cooking breakfast. She seems to only need 1-2 hours of sleep and she's rejuvenated. We often tease her that she has some secret government anti-sleep "potion."

Being the day after Valentine's the breakfast conversation turns to disaster date stories. Julie doesn't mention my potential date in front of the kids, and I'm relieved. I'm not quite ready for more questions from them about Michael. She has the kids laughing hysterically on the cast of characters she's dated. The latest one who wanted her to urinate on him.

"Ew gross." Sandra says. "He's probably a serial killer isn't he?"

"Just a creep." David answers. "Really and he said that on the first date?"

"Yup!" Julie responds. "The first and last date."

I sit at the table and help myself to the spread, laughing with Julie and the kids. Once we finish eating, Julie leaves. She has work to do, and knows I have a project I want to finish. I briefly speak to Michael after she leaves. I'm a bit nervous, but relieved that Michael and I agree not tell the rest of the guys. Well except for John since he was the closest to the both of us, and would eventually figure it out anyway. Michael picks a seafood restaurant that was located on the water. I ask if we could meet at the restaurant, I don't want my kids seeing me going out on a date. Also, if the date is going absolutely nowhere, it is much easier to exit a restaurant and get in your car, than have to endure a torturous ride home with the individual.

I finish my project rather quickly and have enough time to take a relaxing bubble bath. While in the tub, I am able to clear my mind of any worries I have. While getting dressed, I blast my "strong woman" CD. It is a CD Julie and I made in high school: Aretha Franklin, Big Mama Thornton, Cyndi Lauper, Joan Jett, Whitney, Janet Jackson, Pat Benatar, Salt N Pepa, Jody Watley, Madonna etc. If she's a woman that in our minds has overcome adversity, and paved the way, she's on there. Some get on because they have sassy songs. It helps to put me in "the mood" and relaxes me even more. I decide I'm taking it in the car with me, I might need to channel one or two of these women.

I leave the house early and hit almost no traffic. The hostess shows me to the table and I order a martini. I like arriving early. I have picked up a few pointers from Julie on reading body language. Arriving early, allows me to study him as he enters the room, and look for "clues" about his personality.

Michael arrives as I have my first sip of martini. He appears to like to be early as well. When I see him, I almost choke. He looks absolutely amazing. He is dressed in a black sweater and pants that compliment his complexion. I can barely focus. He is extremely confident. As he gets closer to my personal space, I can smell his cologne. WOW! I have never smelled any man like this. It was like the scent was custom blended for him. He has a bunch of irises in a vase. I feel like fainting. Pull it together I tell myself. Channel Ms. Aretha Franklin, calling Ms. Aretha Franklin, I need you now!

He leans in and kisses me on the check. I must be every shade of red right now.

"I hope you weren't waiting long." He says.

"No actually, I just got here." I reply.

We sit down at our table which is a large cozy booth. The conversation is very easy and free-flowing. He asks me if I enjoy working for myself, I tell him I love it because I've always enjoyed writing, and it gave me the flexibility to be with my children and make sure whatever activity they wanted to participate in, they could. The technical side came from growing up in a house full of men. He tells me he decided to go into counseling because he enjoys working with kids and someone close to him committed suicide. I feel like I could tell him anything, and listen to him for hours.

Somehow, our hands meet during the appetizers. Neither one of us pull away. Then we gradually begin to feed one another. I'm not too sure what I was eating. I was trying to maintain my composure every time he caressed my hand, fed me, or moved my hair behind my ear. Ms. Aretha, please don't leave me now. My senses are on overload. It could be all those months of flirting buildup, or maybe the seafood, but my body was screaming to pounce on him. After dessert, he somehow manages to grab my feet and proceeds to give me a foot massage under the table. At which point I had to sing "Respect" to myself at least twice so I wouldn't lose it.

"You know," he starts "I was attracted to you the first time I saw you. John told me there would be a widow at the games, and you were hands off, but not to worry, that I could still curse and belch in front of you. I thought you were going to be this old, dowdy-looking woman. I was floored when I saw how hot you were."

Wow! Thanks John! I think to myself. "Yeah, the guys are a bit overprotective since technically they were my husband's friends first. You are actually the first guy that came to a game that I found attractive, so I never knew what they told the new guys."

"That's good to hear." Michael laughs. "Well, as much as I don't want this night to end, I do have to be up early for work."

"I have basketball mom duties tomorrow unfortunately as well. But I enjoyed myself, and would like to see you again." Ha! I think too myself. How's that for strong confident woman?

"I also would like that very much. When are you free again?"

"Weeknights are usually pretty hectic for me with two kids in sports, and one that just recently added drama to her resume. Weekends are usually better."

"How about Friday and Saturday?"

"It's a date!" I respond. Ugh! That sounds cliché, I need to come up with something else.

Michael slides out the both and helps me out. He grabs my valet ticket and holds my hand as he escorts me towards the door. Before we make it to the door, he stops in a remote and dark part of the restaurant. He spins around, and asks "is it okay if I give you a good…"

I lean in and plant one on his lips. He doesn't seem to object, as he pulls me closer. I'm usually not so aggressive. Actually I'm never this aggressive. We are in a super dark spot of the restaurant, and it is almost empty. It is a kiss that lasts for what seems like hours. It is beyond intense – so intense that I knew I would be sleeping with him soon. I wanted to rip his clothes off there. However, as aggressive as I was feeling, I'm not quite ready to be an exhibitionist. The public kiss was my limit.

We part and I see that he has both a look of bewilderment and satisfaction on his face. I'll take it! We walk outside not saying a word to each other. As the valet pulls my car up, I gave him another kiss, this time, a quick peck. I wish him a good night, and promise that I would text him as soon as I arrive home safely.

I made the mistake of not putting in my aggressive woman CD on the drive home. A wave of guilt overwhelms me. I have never felt passion like that in a kiss before – not even with my husband. I feel so guilty, that I knew I had to have a three way conversation with my friends as soon as I got home, well I'll text Michael first, then I'll call them. I should be home by midnight, but they are probably wide-awake, and probably talking about me.

Chapter 8

"Girlfriend! It's 12:00 am! Why is the date over so soon?" Julie yells into the phone.

"Can you hold so I call Rob?" I reply.

"No need, I have him on the other line. I'll conference him in. You know we were talking about you." She laughs. "We have tons of questions - full disclosure please!"

"Can I just tell my story?" I don't know why I bother asking, I know what their response will be.

They ignore me and start with their questions. "Is he a psychologist or psychiatrist, can he get us pills?"

"More psychologist. I think more social worker. Not sure, will find out." I reply.

"Oh nice, so he is in touch with his emotions."

"How tall, wait, does he have a Facebook profile?"

"OMG! Rob, check him out, he's gorgeous. Does he have a brother? What kind of therapy, because he can cure all problems I'm sure." Julie laughs.

"Oh don't act like you don't have a satellite pointed at his house right now zeroing in on him Julie." Rob teases.

"Was he a gentleman?"

"Yes, beyond so." I sigh.

"Ok, good. Have all his teeth?" Rob asks. He has a thing about teeth. Did not matter what he looked like, if a man has nice teeth, he has a chance with him.

"Yes, he has all his teeth, and he gave me a foot massage under the table." I answer.

"That little freak!" Julie laughs into the phone. "I'm so jealous right now."

I answered all their questions, not like I really have a choice in the matter. It is something that we did with each other whenever there was a new potential. This one seemed more promising, as it has been some time since one of us dated someone who had been "prescreened."

"Did you at least give him a good night kiss since you got a foot massage?" Rob asks.

"A foot massage could have allowed him second base." Julie jokes.

"Yes, he got a good night kiss. It was beyond amazing. If you are finished your questions, I can finally tell you my issue. I feel a bit guilty. I have never kissed someone like that, and well he has a girlfriend. So technically I'm a potential for him. I just felt the guilt building up as I was driving home."

"Guilt for what?" Rob shouts in the phone. "Honey, you

have lived most of your life for other people for so long, it is time to do you! Guilty of his girlfriend? Please! You've seen your brothers, and friends dating other people. It's the nature of the beast. Sometimes the potentials become real partners, and sometimes they don't. He's not married to her, and if she was doing everything correctly, there would be NO YOU. In this day and age who waits for a guy over 2 years without an engagement ring?"

"Uh, question?" Julie interjects. "What isn't she doing correctly? Can you find out? I mean it is known that he is dating someone else, you should be allowed to ask. I hope you continue to date others as well. Don't put all your chickens in a basket. Serial date, and find out where his head is. Now! What's his full name and date of birth?"

"No need for you to check him out Julie. John has vouched for him, that's enough for now." I answer.

"If you say so, but if you want me to check him out…" She retorts.

"Yes, I will let you know." I interrupt.

Julie was right. She did have a valid point. Why you would string someone along, and date other people? Maybe they had an open relationship? That would make things easier for me, it would allow me to see other people, and figure out why his kiss seems to have my head spinning. First thing tomorrow morning, I will speak with Michael, better to establish where we see things going now instead of confusion later.

Chapter 9

I wake early the next day with a smile on my face. I replay the date in my mind over and over again. I even let out a content sigh. This was hugely embarrassing. I am usually not one that is sold so easy, for the simple reason of growing up watching my brothers date. But this one seems different somehow. Would he actually make it pass my weeding out point to meet my kids? Speaking of my kids, they will be up soon and we'll have to pick up members of the basketball team. I decide it is a perfect time to call Michael.

"Hello." His voice is a little gruff, but very sexy. ARGH!! Focus, stay focused.

"Hi Michael, it is Amanda. Is this a good time?"

"For you, I will make time. Did you enjoy your night? I had one of the best nights of my life." He answers.

"Yes, I did have a fabulous time, thank you." He'd probably think I was a complete loser if he knew how much I really enjoyed it. Focus Amanda, focus. "Would it be okay if we meet this afternoon or evening and talk?"

"Sure, how long do you need. I get off at 6:00 today. We can meet any time after? I just can't stay long. I promised my family I'd go to the movies with them at 9:00. Just text me where and when you want to meet."

"That sounds great!" Oh God, did my heart just flutter? "I will see you then." Good I had time to refocus and plan what I was going to say.

Sandra enters my room, just as I hang up the phone. "Mom, we should be ready to go in an hour."

"Ok sweetie!" I respond, pleased for the distraction. I pull myself out of bed, jump in the shower, and put on my "Mom" hat.

Chapter 10

Rap music blasting, three boys in the van, one more to pick up, my cell phone buzzes. Sandra picks it up. "It's a text from Aunt Julie. She said she has a change in plans and will be at the game."

"Ok, thanks babe." I reply. I am relieved Julie will be there. I can practice different scenarios with her, so I will be prepared for the conversation with Michael. Since it is my turn behind the table at the cake sale, she'll also make the time go by faster.

We pull in the school parking lot, and I see Julie's car. Somehow whenever she arrives first, there always seems to be a parking spot next to her whenever I arrive.

I park, and the boys exit the car. Sandra stays behind to wait for Julie and me.

"Sandy, if you want to be with your friends, I'll help your mom behind the table."

"Thanks Aunt Julie! You are the best!" Sandra takes off behind her brother, as Julie and I head towards the school.

"Besides," she says as if she's still speaking to Sandra, "your mom wants to talk about Michael some more."

"Am I THAT obvious?" I sigh.

"Oooh yes! You got it bad! But I can tell there's some stuff you want to still chat about. Who knows you better than me? Who knows me better than you?"

We link arms and head into the gym. "So what do you want to go over? Still that guilty feeling crap?" She asks.

"Yes and no, not so much the guilty feeling, but I'm confused about his feelings for his girlfriend. Does he really like her? Why is he dating other people if he's been with her for so long? I also need to know if he has any guilty feelings."

"Good questions! If he hadn't been prescreened, I'd tell you to run for your life. Don't look back. He's a self-centered, deranged, sick-in-the-head bastard. On one hand, the guys I'm sure have checked him out. On the other hand, serial killers have been known to hide their evil intent by being charming individuals."

"Oh great! Thanks! Like I don't have enough to worry about right now." I pout.

"Listen Mandy, you haven't been on a date or had a potential in what, a while? The good news is that he is prescreened, and you've known him as a friend first, so he hopefully at least cares for you in that sense. Unless he is a self-centered, deranged, sick-in-the-head bastard. And if he is, I'll make sure he regrets it." Julie states giving me her "I'm just kidding, but maybe I'm not" smile.

Julie and I do table setup, and wait for the crowd. This should be a busy one as we're playing our rivals. It is easy being behind the table with Sandra or Julie. Sandra being a popular student and one who respects everyone always draws people to her. Julie is a charmer, and often times has gotten people to purchase their own donations. I just have to sit and smile every now and then and count the money. We always sell out at halftime. This game doesn't seem to be any different. With Julie doing most of the talking, I can mentally go over in my mind the questions I'm going to ask Michael. By halftime we sell out as predicted, hand in the cash box, and sit in the bleachers to watch the rest of the game. It was a close game, but David scores the winning basket as the clock ticks down.

I am temporarily relieved of my basketball mom duties as several students want to walk over to the local diner to celebrate. I told my kids that was fine, however I needed confirmation from the other boy's parents. As I wait for a phone calls from their parents, I decide it is a good time to text Michael. I glance at my watch, 5:45. That should give me enough time to talk to Michael. I text him to meet me at a tea house that is in the area.

Julie gives me a huge bear hug and wishes me luck before she jumps in her car. "I can sit a table or two over if you like?" She teases.

"No, I think I got this. I have our strong woman CD in the car. But thanks!"

I sit in my car for 15 minutes to make sure all the kids I'm in charge of go in the diner and don't come out. Lucky for me they get a booth by the window. Once I am satisfied that it appears no one is going to slip out, I head over to the tea house.

Chapter 11

I arrive first, order a chai latte, and get a booth in the darkest part of the restaurant. I am the only customer here. Probably because of the big game. Anyone who is "out" is probably at the diner celebrating. Michael arrives with a bouquet of gerbera daisies.

"Are you giving me flowers in separate bouquets now?" I tease.

"Well I really didn't think they made an attractive bouquet with your other favorites after I ordered it. So I figured I would separate them." He laughs. "How was the game?"

"Awesome! David scored the winning basket."

He slides into my side of the booth and pulls me in for a deep kiss. We parted when we sense the waitress arriving. I don't think she saw us as the table is strategically placed so you can see everywhere, but thanks to some plants, you have a good 5 second recovery time.

"Can I get you anything?" She asks. Michael orders a green tea while caressing my hand, and we decide to split a slice of carrot cake. I'm starting to swoon, and if I don't get this conversation going soon, I won't be able to ask my questions. Once she leaves, I gather my strength and "go for it."

"Thank you for coming. I just needed to ask you a couple of things. Just to make sure we are on the same page." I begin.

"No problem, I am an open book for you. Fire away." He responds while kissing my fingers.

Ok, he does not seem nearly as nervous as I am right now. How do I get the questions out of my mouth and sound coherent? Especially with him kissing my fingers? I'll try not to have too much eye contact with him. Only towards the end of the question.

"Well, I really enjoyed myself last night. I have not had that much fun, or felt that comfortable with anyone in a long time. But I need to know. Do you have any regrets about last night?" I get the first question out. Score one for the breathless lady.

"Regrets? No, why would I have any regrets? Do you have any regrets?" He asks, showing concern.

"Well, no, I reply. But I am not the one in a serious relationship."

"Ah that. Well, honestly, I am not sure where that is going. I'll be honest with you. I have dated other women before you. And well there are a lot of problems with my relationship. It is at an extremely boring point right now, and I try speaking to her about it, but she is pretty complacent about it. The sex has pretty much disappeared. Plus she is Christian, so that has been getting in the way one time too many times."

"What do you mean because she is Christian?"

"She's Catholic. Well for one, it took us a whole year to finally have sex. Her parents do not know we are dating, only her brother. He accepts me, her parents don't."

I silently sighed. Ah yes, the "religious people." The people who pick and choose what parts of their religion they want to follow. Hello? Honor they mother and father, it is a Ten Commandment. Also, there should be no premarital sex for all Christian religions. Sex for Catholics was only to procreate. Let's not even get into the rhythm method. Don't get me wrong, there are those that are true and follow the laws of their religion and lead their life accordingly. Although I am no longer a religious person, those that "walk the walk" have my highest respect.

"So you're just looking for a sex toy?" I ask.

"Oh God no! The other women I've dated, I had no connection to. I felt nothing for them. Yeah, I could've had sex with them, but I didn't. Well with one of them I did, but I hated every minute of it. You're the first woman who I've felt comfortable with, and who I feel I can be myself with. I know we've only been on one date, but I've enjoyed each and every conversation we've had. Even at the poker games. You're gorgeous, funny, kind, secure. I've never met anyone like you. I'd be lying if I said I wasn't attracted to you physically, but it goes way beyond that."

Ok. So I felt I had enough information. For now.

"Well do you have any questions for me?" I ask.

"No." He replies. "I just would really like to kiss you some more."

"Fire away." I respond.

Like two teenagers we "make out" in the restaurant until my cell phone buzzes. I have a special ring tone for my kids.

"My kids." I say as I pull away. "They must be ready for me to pick them up."

Sandra: Ready in 15 minutes. Thnx!

Michael pays the bill and walks me to my car. We had one more deeply intense kiss before he opens my car door. "I can't wait for next Friday." He says as he kisses me softly on my forehead.

"Me too." I get in the car and he closes the door. I focus on my kids, and it helps clear the mind. I start my car, blow him a kiss, and pull out the parking lot. I am relieved we met in a public place or who knows what might have happened? If we had not met in a public place, we probably would have ended with both of us naked and horizontal, or upside down, or oooh, focus on driving. This man awakens emotions in me that have been dormant for years. We should probably have that sex talk sometime soon – really soon.

Chapter 12

I arrive home within an hour of completing my basketball mom duties. I grab my phone out my bag so I can charge it. I had thrown it in my bag once I arrived at the diner. There was a text from Michael.

Michael: Thank you for our talk. I miss you. I want to be an open book for you, so feel free to ask me anything you need to.

Okay. So he follows up. But sure most guys do in the beginning, before they sleep with you. So I will not be impressed so easily. I should respond to his text, let's see. Show strong interest, but not too needy.

Me: Thank you for being honest with me. I appreciate it. I look forward to seeing you again soon. ☺

Oh crap! Maybe I shouldn't have sent the smiley face? This texting is all too new to me. I do it with my kids, and friends. So who cares if I say or do something stupid with them? This texting sweet nothings is a new phenomenon for me. I believe I saw it on the news – sexting? I also don't know all the texting abbreviations, I hope he doesn't use them.

My phone vibrates me out of my thoughts. It is John.

John: So wasssssup boo? How did it go? Did you kiss him at least? Slip some tongue? Heavy duty fondling?

Who ever said men don't like to gossip? I'm not ready to tell John anything, and I won't.

Me: Sorry, but you know I don't kiss and tell. Whatever information you need, you will have to get from him.

John: Yeah thnx! I got the same response from him.

Wow! That's interesting. I know from my brothers that guys always talk about dates, unless they are REALLY interested in the girl. Could Michael be THAT interested in me? Breathe, focus Amanda.

BZZZZZZZZZZZZ, another text. From Michael.

Michael: Friday seems like years away. I would love to see you sooner.

Me: What is going to happen when we do see each other?

Michael: Good question, what do you think we are going to do? When we see each other?

Excellent, he feels the chemistry too! He is answering my question with a question. Typical guy thing to do when they are not quite sure how their answer will be received.

Hmmm, now would probably be a good time to get the pre-sex stuff out of the way, if I worded it correctly. Got it!

Me: So technically we've been dating for close to a year now. Do you think that kissing is all we'll be doing?

I smile as I hit send. I put the ball back in his court. He got what I meant right away.

Michael: Not that I don't want to, but do you think we are ready for the next step?

Oh! He's good! But not that good. I can play the male question game with the best of them.

Me: Do you honestly think if we are in a place with no restrictions, we will stick to just kissing?

Michael: Yes.

Well that was an excitement killer. Okay either he is the perfect gentlemen, or just knows the right things to say. Too early to tell. Ok, let's kill the moment even more and throw out the STD question.

Me: Sorry to kill the mood, but when was your last STD test, and what was the outcome?

I think I could get used to this sexting. You can just throw anything out there, and not have to worry about seeing the other person's reaction.

Michael: You're not killing the mood. I was tested just last month. The program I work for makes me do it. I was clear of everything. When was yours?

Me: Six months ago, there hasn't been anyone in a while. I am clear of everything. I can get you copies. I actually make sure to get tested for stuff every six months. When you have children, you can be neurotic about things.

Michael: No need to see copies, I trust you Do you want to see mine?

Me: No, you may not be much of a poker player, but I trust you. It just seems like we've been dating for a year now, instead of just playing poker. That is why I am wondering if we can just keep things to kissing?

My phone starts ringing, indicating a phone call was coming in. It was Michael.

"Hello." I say trying to keep my cool.

"Sorry for calling so late, but do you care to wager a bet?" He asks.

"Sure what are we going to bet?"

"How about loser gives the other one a full-body massage?"

"Deal!" I respond.

"Excellent, I've been tense lately. I'm going back in the movies, I will speak with you tomorrow."

So he is willing to hold out. Interesting. Maybe he is not as interested in me as much as I was in him. Maybe he is the rare man that does not think about sex all day and night? I have heard of search creatures. Did not know they really existed. Or maybe since it has been a while since I have had a male partner my sexual desires were higher than his.

Bzzzzzzzzzzzzzzz. Another text. This one from Michael.

Michael: I can't wait until Friday. When can I see you again? Are you free tomorrow?

Me: Tomorrow is no good. My kids have practice. How about the day after tomorrow? They're going on an overnight trip with the school.

Michael: Good! I will see you then! Anyplace in particular you would like to go?

Me: No, there are really no movies out I want to see. Why don't you come here? We could rent some movies? I can cook for us. You can come any time after 5:00.

Michael: That works for me! I will see you then. I am looking forward to it.

Me: Me too. It's a date.

Ugh! Mental note, come up with something clever to say to Michael when responding to his plans.

Chapter 13

The next morning, I wake alarmed. I have nothing sexy or any matching lingerie to wear. Yes, it has been THAT long since I have been with a man intimately. I have to schedule a quick run to the lingerie store. I wonder what is his favorite color? Wait! Did someone mention he was is a fraternity, I giggle to myself. Maybe I should wear those colors. Which frat was it? Ugh! I cannot remember to save my life. Maybe I will just see what is on sale. It is a good thing he is coming over in the evening; it gives me more time to organize my kids and find something to wear. I should also figure out what to cook.

I should call Julie. No, I'll text her in case she is in some important meeting.

Me: Hey Julie, no drive-bys tomorrow, Michael is coming over. Any suggestions on lingerie color?

I probably won't get a response from her until later. If she is in her office, she won't answer her personal phone.

The rest of the day and the next one seemed to last 6 months mentally. Planning a scrumptious meal, running my kids around and going to the lingerie store only seem to drag out the time. Julie did return my text before my trip to the mall.

Julie: Something green. It's your color. Hooch! ☺

I was in luck. I found a green lacey set that was on sale. It was an out of season color or something or other. Men don't pay attention to fashion seasons. It was 75% off, score!

With all of the running around I was doing, I forgot to be nervous. That is until Michael finally rings my bell at 6:00. I feel a slight churn in my stomach. I slowly exhale and tell myself that I can do this.

I open the door, and was immediately scooped up in his arms for a long, passionate kiss. If this keeps up, I would probably commit any crime he asks me to.

"Did you miss me?" I whisper.

"Very much so, I promise to show you how much. Are your kids here?" He questions.

"Not to worry, we have the house to ourselves. Shall we eat now?" I ask in between kisses.

"I'm not thinking about food right now." He answers with his lips against the nape of my neck.

I shock myself by letting out a low, throaty groan. That seems to be all the encouragement he needs. He picks me up and carries me to the living room, where he gently lays me down on the couch, and then lays down on top of me.

Not sure who pulls off whose clothes first, but all of our clothes end on the floor rather quickly. He is beyond masterful with his mouth and caresses. I finally manage to tell him that we had should move to the bedroom, I have condoms and they are in there.

"I have my own, I prefer a certain brand." He states.

The walk to the bedroom takes longer than it should. We could not break our lip lock, nor could we stop caressing each other. We make it to my room and continue the kissing and caressing on top of my bed. It is obvious he knows what he is doing. He expertly kisses, sucks and caresses my breasts, and I finally reach my point where could take no more, I had to have him. I beg him to put on a condom; I see the hesitation in his face. There is no way I'm going back now. I am too heated to go back. I need to be the aggressor that I hear guys say they like so much.

"I'm so wet for you right now, I need you inside me." I purr.

Talk about a bad porno line, but it works. The hesitation melts away from his face, and he immediately puts the condom on. What happens the rest of the night is amazing. I didn't think I could orgasm so many times. We go through a box and a half of Trojan magnums. The more we have of each other, the more insatiable for each other we become.

After several hours we eventually pass out in each other's arms, panting, sweaty, giddy, and weak but satiated. We nap for a time, and then stomach hunger kicks in by early morning. I would've insisted on eating dinner had I know we were going to have a marathon sex session. I glance at the clock. 3:00 am. Dinner is probably out of the question, perhaps an early breakfast is in order.

Chapter 14

I roll over and catch him wide awake and staring at me. I give him my best seductive smile, or at least I think I did. "How about I go make us some breakfast in bed? Then shower? You can stay here and watch TV if you like."

"Well I kind of have a thing about eating in the bed, it leaves crumbs." He replies. "So how about we shower, and then I help you make breakfast?"

"That works for me!" I reply, probably a little too enthusiastically.

After some heavy duty kissing and caressing in the shower, we finally manage to finish. We walk to the kitchen wearing towels.

"What time are your kids coming back?" He asks, seeming troubled.

"Don't worry, if you want to drop the towel, they won't be back until tomorrow." I respond with a devilish grin.

"I just wanted to make sure. I would not want to meet them

like this. I would rather make a good first impression."

"Good point." I respond. "So I make a mean French Toast. I make it with challah bread. It is usually really filling, but I think some scrambled eggs and bacon on the side are in order, as I'm feeling very ravenous for some reason."

Michael laughs and replies "I'll let you decide. I feel I'm in pretty good hands. Besides I want to make sure I'll be well taken care of in my old age."

As I pull out the ingredients to start breakfast, a thought pops into my head. Was what I said to start the most amazing sex of my life too much? I am standing in my kitchen in a towel with a man who is also dressed in a towel. There is no more room for modestly at this point. I can just ask him.

"Uh, Michael." I start. "I am really sorry if I forced you into something which you may not have wanted to do. I was just very turned on by you, mentally and physically, and I…"

"Amanda, you did not force me into doing anything that I did not want to do. Trust me, I feel the same way. I only hesitated because I was nervous. I just wanted to make sure I pleased you in every way possible. I have been dreaming about this since I first met you. But the guys are VERY protective of you. I had to go through an intense interview, and John had to vouch for my character."

"Just what I need! Four more brothers." I groan.

We both laugh and he stands up and pulls me in his arms and we start kissing. I somehow manage to pull myself away. "You are very dangerous. A girl can forget she has to eat food with you."

He laughs and replies. "I will let you finish preparing, just tell me how I can help, so I can get back to kissing you."

So I give him the eggs and tell him to start cracking and

scrambling. We prepare breakfast in silence. But it was a comfortable silence. No one felt forced to say anything. We finally sit down to eat and Michael pauses.

"Is something wrong?" I ask.

"Don't Christians say grace before you eat?" He replies.

"Yeah, well I am really not that religious. I do the grace thing with my kids sometimes, but it is really not a necessity for me. I hope that is okay with you."

He laughs. "Why would I mind? I am just trying to impress you."

"You don't have to try." I respond. "You already have. The proof is in the fact that you are in my house and I made you breakfast."

"And I am very grateful."

We spend the next couple of hours talking about our goals, ambitions, and sports. After we finish eating, he loads the dishes in the dish washer, and we go back to my room for another kissing session. While watching the movie, my phone rings. I check my caller ID to make sure it is not my kids. I see it is Amy, a former client who has become a dear friend.

"Amanda babes! I met the most awesome guy for you. I told him how great you are, and showed him a picture. He's dying to meet you. So call me and I'll set it up. Hope all is well! My love to the kids!"

"You are not going to call her back are you?" Michael asks. "I don't think I'd be comfortable with it."

Ummmmm, am I missing something? Maybe he is joking. So I roll over to face him. No, there is no sarcasm in his face. He is serious.

"It is just a blind date." I respond. "None of those ever work out. Aren't you still with someone?"

"Yes, but I don't want to share you." He responds.

WHOA! He doesn't want to share me? Is he serious? "I have tons of friends and colleagues who love me and who think I am a fabulous person and I should have someone in my life." I explain. "They are constantly trying to set me up with someone. For me not to go out with the guy, would upset the people who love me."

"Well, do you really want to meet someone? Or are you just going through the motions?" He asks.

"I think everyone wants to be with someone. I really do not put high expectations on blind dates as it sets you up for disappointment. I just go out on them, and see how things flow."

"I am not sure if I am comfortable with that. I am very old-fashioned."

Is he serious? If he was old-fashioned, wouldn't he be married by now?

"Isn't that a bit hypocritical? I am after all, sharing you."

"Yes, but I haven't had sex with her since we started kissing." Michael answers.

I wanted to ask if he wasn't having sex with her, then what did she think he was doing in his spare time? Obviously, someone who goes through a box and a half of condoms in a night is a sexual and passionate person. Perhaps I shouldn't ask that question now. I don't want our first fight to be over a blind date and what his girlfriend is thinking. That will be filed in the mental storage cabinet and asked later.

Before I could form another question, Michael lets out a sigh. "I guess I see your point, but I still don't like it."

He gently caressed my mouth with his, and I took that as a sign to drop the subject. So I turn back around to watch the movie and pull him closer to me.

At 10:00 that night he decides to leave because he has to get up early the next day. We had finished off the second box of condoms several hours earlier. We share one last passionate kiss before he leaves.

I am too worn out to change my linen. As I pass out in my bed, I exhale a content sigh. I get a whiff of his cologne and thought I may not wash my linen for a couple of days. I run over the day's activities, including our first argument. I am relieved we had a proper adult discussion about it, and it was not a screaming, insulting drag-out fight. Could he also be the only man left that likes to discuss his displeasures rationally? I have it bad, I have to admit to myself, but we are going to need to work on his jealousy issues. I fall asleep rather early, still exhausted from the previous night's activities.

Chapter 15

My phone rings, and I jump up startled, hoping it is not something with my kids. The caller ID says it is Michael.

"Hello." I answer trying to sound seductive.

"Hi boo, I just wanted to let you know that I had the most amazing night of my life. Thank you. I can't wait to see you again. I feel like I just can't spend one day with you."

"Me too, I miss you already." I respond ignoring the fact he called me boo. We'll have to talk about that later, don't want to ruin the moment now and perhaps start another argument. Also filed in the mental cabinet. One of the most important rules about serial dating is not to let yourself be called a "pet name." Chances are he is using the same name with the other girls he's dating.

"You have me Friday and Saturday. Oh! My kids are actually going to visit my brother in California for spring break. You could have me the entire week."

"Excellent! We will definitely have to plan something the week of Spring Break. I am looking forward to this weekend."

"I am too! What are we going to do?" I respond.

"Oh, I think we do better when we wing it. However, let's see what we can come up with tomorrow. Get some rest. I miss you."

"I miss you too." I respond.

I hang up smiling. The phone starts ringing again. It is my brother Billy. "Mandy did I wake you?"

"No, I'm wide awake I respond."

"Since the kids are coming Spring Break, you should come too." I wonder if I'll be in my 70's and my brothers will treat me like the baby. They always assume I have nothing to do. Well I probably wouldn't have anything to do, but now I have Michael.

"Thanks Billy, but I have plans."

"Really? With Julie and Rob? They can come too."

Ah, yes. I love how married people always assume if you're single, you have no plans, and you can make them at the drop of a dime. Yes married people we have lives too! Sometimes we're busier than you!

"No, I have a huge project I want to finish. I was planning on doing it that week since I won't have to drive the kids around." It is the partial truth. I decide to leave out the Michael part. Don't want to mention him yet.

I hang up the phone, and inhale Michael's scent in my bed. Wait! I sit up in bed. We're spending the whole week together? Why isn't he spending time with his girlfriend? That's interesting. I recline back into my pillows. I have every right to ask why he's not spending a week with her since he is jealous of me, but on second thought, I rather not know. He will be with me and that's all the matters.

I eventually close my eyes. Blissful thoughts of Michael form as I inhale his scent from my pillows.

Chapter 16

The next day, I wake at 9:30 am. I am still in a blissful place that makes me somewhat slothful. I roll over in bed to get the phone to return Amy's call. She answers after the first ring.

"Amanda! Babes! I have the perfect guy. I showed him your picture, blah, blah, blah." I tune her out. My thoughts return to Michael. I am glad I work from home and set my own hours. I do not know how I could sit in an office and focus right now. I salute the office workers.

While she is talking I decide to send Michael a text. Rather a sext. I want to say something cute and somewhat risqué. Got it.

ME: Hi sexy, I totally miss you inside me.

I think I love this sexting! You lose your inhibitions. Just put it out there.

I receive an immediate response.

Michael: I totally miss being inside you. I don't think I can wait until Friday.

A big grin appears on my face.

"Amanda! Are you still there?"

Oh yeah! I still have Amy on the phone. "Yes I am still here. Just absorbing everything you're saying. So what are his issues?" I hope she didn't say them already.

"That's the best part! None! He has his own business and he is back in school working on a MBA, and blah, blah, blah, blah…"

Me: What about meeting for a quickie?

Oh! Maybe I should have phrased that differently? I am not complaining about his stamina. I know sometimes things can be misinterpreted via text. Need to send a quick recovery text.

Me: Not that I think there is anything quick about you.

There! That should be a good recovery.

Michael: I didn't want to ask, but I'd love too. Although, I rather take my time with you.

"Awesome!" I text and say out loud at the same time.

"I know right?" Amy responds. I forgot again I was speaking to Amy.

Me: What should I wear? Extra layers so you can take your time?

Michael: I think I like the sound of that! Let me check my work schedule? My place?

Me: Perfect.

"So agreed, I will give him your cell phone number, and have him call you." Amy continues. "He is going to a conference at the end of the week, so I am sure he will want to meet you before then as I showed him your picture and told him how great you are. Let him make the first move."

I sigh. Amy is still old-fashioned. But I should probably meet someone new. Michael has my head spinning. Probably better to meet someone else. It would help me refocus and have a reality check. I do realize I have known him for a year, but this does seem to be moving rather quickly. We end our conversation and I decide to go to my office to work on a project

Chapter 17

I am intensely focused on work and finishing the project, that I do not realize several hours have passed. BZZZZZZZZZZZZZZZZZZZZZZZZZZZ. My phone vibrates indicating another text. I smile as I am sure it is Michael.

Hi Amanda, this is Randy, Amy's friend. She told me I would want to meet you, and she showed me your picture and I agreed.

Well that was fast, but something about his message immediately annoyed me. He couldn't call the first time? Alright, maybe he is shy. No one's perfect, and I include myself in the not being perfect group.

Me: Hi Randy. Amy said you were going to a conference, at the end of the week – you wanted to meet soon? The only night I have free this week is Wednesday. I have activities with my kids the other nights.

My phone vibrates almost immediately. It is Michael. *Changed my mind. I want you to wear something that I will have easy access to – something that will come off quickly.*

Me: No problem. But what are you going to wear? Something I can take off with my teeth, I hope.

Take that! I smile triumphantly.

BZZZZZZZZZ

Wednesday is great. Where do you want to meet?

Huh? Oh! It's Randy. Let me stop texting Michael for a bit and hurry Randy along.

Me: I eat all types of foods and have no allergies or dietary restrictions. Why don't you decide?

Work with me dude! Pick something.

Michael: ROTFL! I will have to think of something.

Randy: No, no, I insist you pick something.

Argh! I have little patience for the indecisive guy. You can totally make a good impression picking the restaurant yourself. It is perfectly fine to ask if I have any food allergies and/or food restrictions. But if you want to start off with bonus points, you pick for the first date.

Me: There is a really good Japanese restaurant on Franklin Avenue. We can go there. I will meet you there at 5:00 pm.

If I have to pick the restaurant, I am picking the time.

Randy: Great! I love sushi. I will see you then.

Whatever dude I say to myself. Hopefully you can crawl out of this hole you dug.

Another buzz. It is Michael. *What are you doing tomorrow at noon? I don't have to go to my evening job, and I'm getting out early for the day one.*

Me: YOU!

Michael: Good answer. Come to my place. I will be waiting for you.

Me: Can't wait.

This is awesome! Although Randy has annoyed me initially, if the date goes poorly, I will probably be riding high from my afternoon quickie, and looking forward to my date on Friday and Saturday. Excellent! I am quite excited as I throw myself back into my project and spend the rest of the evening working.

Chapter 18

Thank God it's Tuesday! I am looking forward to today, my kids come back, and I'm in for an awesome sexual adventure! Plus it is raining! Awesome! I can wear a rain coat, and this new bra and panty set I purchased underneath the coat. I read in Cosmo that the rain coat and bra and panty set at the door was a fantasy for the majority of men. I hope Michael isn't the exception in this case. I "suit up" and jump in the car. I stop and pick up a bouquet of flowers for Michael. He buzzes me into the building, and I walk to his apartment. He is waiting at the door and yanks me into his arms immediately.

He places the flowers on the table as he starts to undo my raincoat. His lets out a deep throaty moan while we are still locked in a kiss, so I know he approves of my outfit choice. He immediately picks me up and carries me to his bedroom. I guess I'll get a tour later – but who cares? There is nothing quick about his quickie. He is completely thorough, and after a couple of hours, we pass out in each other's arms.

"I loved that outfit." He whispers in my ear.

"I am glad you approve. It took me some time to pick it out. I wanted you to be impressed."

"It worked." He responds. "You are staying the night aren't you?"

"I can't. My kids come home today. Mommy duties."

"Can I ask you a question?" Michael starts. "What would happen if we became pregnant?"

That's an odd question, I think to myself. "Well, if I get you pregnant, we should keep the baby. We could probably make a lot of money and retire early."

Michael laughs and gives me a couple of quick kisses.

"Well I really didn't give it much thought." I continue. "It is not like I'm trying to get pregnant. I am a little too old to be running to some clinic because of our stupid mistake. I would just keep the baby, and you wouldn't have to worry about anything."

"I wouldn't want you to get rid of the baby." He responds. "I would want you to keep the baby, and I wouldn't abandon you. I was just imagining how amazing the baby would look. And how amazing the baby would be. Are you sure you can't stay the night? Sorry I'm being selfish."

I laugh. "It is okay, but I'm sure I can't stay. I have to make sure my kids are well fed when they return. Don't worry, you will have me all to yourself this weekend, and spring break. Rob is taking my kids to some athletic conference or other. Now I have a question for you. Wouldn't me having a baby present some problems for you?"

"No, no problems for me. What is the worst that could happen? Nothing! I can totally handle any situation." He pauses and appears to be mulling something. "I like the sound of having you to myself for an entire weekend." He says while pulling me in for a kiss. His kisses send the usual surges through my entire body. Surges that I never tire of feeling.

I can feel a coldness on my lips when he stops abruptly and pulls away. "Hey, did you make a date? Your blind date from Amy?"

"I did, he sounds annoying, but it is on Thursday." I reply.

"That's good news for me." He says, pulling me back in for another long and passionate kiss.

My thoughts of my kids being home soon help me pull myself away from Michael. I had already made a lasagna and dessert just in case they were hungry. I had plenty of time to get home and shower.

"I should go." I say leaning in for a kiss. "I don't think I could ever get tired of your kisses. You are an amazing kisser."

Michael chuckles. "I am just following your lead."

I get home with an hour to spare. I jump in the shower and quickly change. Sandra and David arrive together both stating how stuffed they are and if I had any dessert.

We sit down to eat and go over each other's day. My day of course was not as detailed as theirs. "Mom you need to get out more, what's the point of working from home? We appreciate you cooking for us, but have some fun." Sandra states.

"We'll see" I reply. If you only knew little one, I think to myself.

The doorbell rings, and David gets up to answer the door. He comes in with a bouquet of flowers. "Michael again? Does this guy own a florist? Have you even gone out with him yet?"

"Cut her some slack." Sandra defends me. "I think it is reassuring when a man sends flowers."

I grab the card from David. "I don't go snooping in your stuff. I would hope that you would do the same for me." I tease.

I read the card. "I miss you and look forward to seeing you again."

I see Sandra and David giggling. Urgh! I'm smiling aren't I? "I am still your mother. Show some respect. Let's drop it."

David changes the subject back to the retreat, and we spend the rest of our meal on topics other than Michael. After dessert, we individually get ready for bed. I close my eyes and dream of Michael and the afternoon we shared.

Chapter 19

The next morning I wake early to fix breakfast. I'm not sure what they ate while they were away, but I want to make sure they have full stomachs going back to school. Over breakfast I tell them I have an appointment at 6:00 and I see them giving each other knowing smiles. I choose to ignore it.

The day passes quickly and I reach the restaurant 10 minutes early. I consider this late, but I'm lucky that he isn't there.

I get a table and order a drink. I finish off my martini and glance at my watch. He is 10 minutes late. Not a good sign. So I order another martini and wait a few more minutes.

BZZZZ. This must be him texting me. I pull out my phone. It is Michael.

Michael: I hope you have a good time tonight.

Me: Do you really mean that?

Michael: Actually I don't. I hope you have a miserable time, and you think about me the whole time.

So far I am having a miserable time. I hate lateness on all levels, whether it is a date, client, or friends. I do not mind lateness if there is a legitimate reason. I will give him the benefit of the doubt, until I meet him. I order shu mai and glance at my watch once they arrive. Now he is 30 minutes late. I should probably send him a text.

Me: Hi Randy, it is Amanda, I just wanted to make sure you are okay.

Randy: I'm outside now.

Me: I'm in a black and white shirt, and I am sitting on the right side of the restaurant.

Maybe he was saving a family from a burning building? Or maybe he was just stuck in bad traffic? Either way, I need an reason for the lateness.

In walks a tall, lanky man. He walks with a certain air of confidence, or arrogance, not quite sure. Time will tell. I go over Julie's checklist in my head. He walks over to the table and sits down.

"Hi Amanda, oh good you ordered appetizers for us." He immediately reaches over and grabs a shu mai.

Well, I guess I will not be receiving an apology for his lateness. So he failed the manners section of the test, I'll try and help out with some extra credit questions, and we'll see where this goes.

"Did you hit any traffic or have problems finding the place?" I ask.

"Oh no! I found it perfectly."

Maybe he is not understanding why I am asking. It happens. Men and women do think on different levels. It is times like this when I wonder if I say what is really on my mind, if I would be considered rude. I would really like to yell: "Hey dork! You're late! An explanation would be nice. "

Perhaps I should ask an essay question? One that will get him to open up and talk some more. The lateness will just have to be ignored at this point. "So Amy tells me you own your own business? What do you do?"

"I do real estate." He responds. More silence.

Well to be fair, he is answering my questions.

"How long have you been doing real estate, how is it going in this economy?"

"I'm good!" He responds.

Annnnnnnnnnnd, I'm done. I watch as he shoves the last shu mai in his mouth. The waiter finally takes our order. More silence, but somehow it is not so awkward for me. I sip my drink and thoughts of Michael form in my mind.

After a good 10 minutes he asks "So Amy tells me you are a technical writer? How did you get into that?" Okay, so that question can get him out of a deficit.

"Well I love writing - I've been told by some teachers I was a horrible writer and other teachers have told me I was a strong writer. So it has always amazed me how different people have different views on writing. I grew up in a household of brothers, so I was a bit of a tomboy. I was constantly following behind them, and gained some mechanical skills along the way. I have disassembled and reassembled several bikes, computers, cars, electrical appliances. You name it; I've probably pulled it apart and reassembled it. Technical writing seems to pull it all together. It also allows me time to make sure my kids are involved in every activity they want."

"I hear you about the kids. I totally want a wife who will stay home and take care of the house and kids. My last girlfriend had kids. We just broke up. I thought I was going to marry her, but she met someone else. So you can do the cooking, cleaning, and repairs. Why the heck are you still single?"

At this point I am beginning to wonder why Amy thought we'd be a good match. His ex was probably a smart woman.

"Just waiting for the right one." I respond.

After a few more martinis he begins to talk a mile a minute. It seems he has forgotten I am here, as I have not said anything in the last 20 minutes. It is also blatantly obvious by his stories, that he still has feelings for his ex. The waiter finally puts the bill on our table. I reach for it, as I just want to bolt for the door. Randy beats me to it.

"Oh no, I got it." He puts his credit card in the fold, and hands it to the waiter. As soon as the waiter brings the holder back and Randy signs for the bill, I stand up.

"Randy, it was nice meeting you, thanks for dinner."

"Sure, text me when you get in, so I know you are safe."

Humph. If you were that concerned, shouldn't you walk me to my car? I kiss him on the cheek. I doubt we will ever have a love connection; hell, we won't even have a friendship connection. We have absolutely nothing in common, and he is boring as hell. I will need to have a talk with Amy. What did she see exactly? The good news is that I'm only ten minutes from home. It was a waste of makeup application night. I think to myself as I pull in my driveway. I take a quick hot shower and climb in bed.

Chapter 20

I wake early to hear my phone buzzing, instead of the alarm. I forgot to turn it off before I got in bed. I grab my phone and look at the time. It is 3:00 in the morning! It is a text from Michael.

Michael: I can't sleep. How was your date?

Really dude!? This isn't even cute anymore. I was about to respond, but realized although he was not able to sleep, I was. I'll let him stew a bit more. I'll tell him when I wake up the date was horrible, but I'll let him worry first. I turn off my phone, calm my nerves and eventually fall back asleep. I wake to the smell of coffee and cinnamon toast. Julie must be here. I climb out of bed and walk into the kitchen. My kids are in the kitchen, but no Julie.

"Did Aunt Julie leave?" I ask.

David and Sandra giggle.

"No." Sandra answers. "We decided to make breakfast for you since you had a hot date last night."

Ahhhh! They think I went out with Michael. They don't

need to know the truth. Besides I get a "free" breakfast out of the deal. They know better to ask personal questions. They seem very proud of their creation. The bacon is extra crispy, and there doesn't appear to be enough flour in the waffles. But the proud mother that I am has me eating the breakfast as if it were a 5 star meal.

"So how are play rehearsals?" I ask Sandra.

"She has to kiss a boy in the play." David interrupts. "I don't know if I'm too happy about that."

Sandra and I both roll our eyes at David. "It's just a play, and it's only a peck! Not like we're exchanging saliva!" Sandra states.

"Is that what you kids are calling kissing now? Exchanging saliva?"

"Well that's what it is Mom!"

"I guess." I respond, thinking perhaps I should change the subject so they don't slip and ask me if I "exchanged saliva" last night. My stomach does a little churn, not sure if it is the food, or the thought of exchanging saliva with Randy.

"HEY! Who made breakfast and didn't invite me?" Julie says as she enters the kitchen.

"We did, Mom had a hot date last night." Sandra giggles.

"I have a limo with a driver outside if you guys want a ride to school." Julie asks. She knows to ignore the hot date comment, at least until the kids leave. The one sure fire way to get them out the door in a hurry is her offer of a limo ride. She gets them from time to time as a job perk. She usually will get the driver to drop "her kids" off to school for an extra tip.

Julie helps herself to the breakfast and pretends like it is the best meal she's had. Once the kids finish up, run outside to the limo, and the limo turns the corner, I grab our plates, and toss the remnants in the garbage.

"How about I make us something else?" I ask.

"I thought you'd never ask." Julie laughs. "The only good thing about that was the love that was put into it. Sooo the hot date, was it with Michael, inquiring minds want to know?" Julie probes.

"In fact, no." I respond. "It was a blind date from Amy. He was late and wouldn't speak in the beginning, but once he started chatting, it was nonstop!"

"Ugh!" Julie groans. "Why do you even bother with her? The guys she has tried to set you up with, have any of them even been decent?"

"Uh, well there was, oooh, ah not him. What about…Ah, yeah. Okay so she has been losing in the setting me up area, but her husband is good catch. I guess it is just wishful thinking that she will find someone with his personality and his unconditional love and support. Oh! You don't think because I had love like that once, I will never get it again do you?"

"Don't be silly!" Julie reacts. "Just because you had one, does not mean you will not get another! Hell! Look at me! Where is my one? I'm tired of men telling me I look too independent. Am I supposed to walk with my shoulders slouched?" Julie stands up to make some coffee. Not that she drinks it, but she makes an awesome pot.

"Do you want me to take you home after we eat?" I question.

"Actually do you mind if I crash here for a couple of hours,

I'm dead tired, and they're doing construction by my house."

"I do mind, if you're asking!" I tease.

"I just didn't know if you were expecting company or not. If you are just text me, and I'll crawl out the window or something. I rather hear the construction than your sex screams."

"You are assuming too much!" I protest.

"Hellooooooooo! It is ME you are talking to!" Julie teases. "You're glowing hotter than a nuclear reactor mama! I know you've gotten some." Julie gives me a smug look that dares me to defy her.

"Well okay, but you don't know if I'm a sexual screamer!"

"Ew! I don't need to have any thoughts about your sexual screams before I go to bed. I need a shower. I'll get the details after I'm rested." Julie blows me a kiss and saunters out the kitchen.

I am left to my thoughts in the kitchen. I should probably return Michael's text. But I'll do it after I load the dish washer.

Once I'm done, I wait another 5 minutes for good measure and I respond to Michael's text.

Me: It was horrible. He was a loser.

Michael: I'm relieved to hear that.

His response was quick considering I made him wait. I guess he really is interested. He just really needs to work through this jealousy issue. I am just going on dates. He has a girlfriend. I decide this is a discussion we need to have soon. There is no reason to move forward if we don't.

Me: I look forward to this weekend. Am I meeting you somewhere? Or are you picking me up? My kids are going away with my friend Rob this weekend.

Michael: Why don't we go to the movies, dinner, and then we'll take it from there? ☺

Me: I like the way that sounds.

If we do movies and dinner, at least I will be able to speak to him about this jealousy situation.

Michael: I'll pick you up at 6.

Me: Sounds good. I'm looking forward to seeing you.

I should probably text something flirty back, but I'm just not in the mood. I head to my office to work on a project. I work for a good four hours before Julie appears.

"Thanks! I needed that rest. I'm energized now and ready for the world." She says as she begins to go through a series of complex yoga stretches. While executing a perfect crane pose she questions me about Michael. "So, how was the sexcursion? When were you going to share the details?"

"Is it that obvious?" I hope David and Sandra can't tell I think to myself.

"Maybe not to David and Sandra." She reassures me. Somehow she always knows to do that. "But to me? Without question. Plus I also know it has been some time since your last one."

"It was amazing. Beyond amazing. I was screaming like I used to with my husband." I sigh.

"No specifics!" Julie protests. "General adjectives will do."

"He had magnum sized condoms. They fit."

Julie makes an impressed face before she laughs. She once dated a guy who insisted on magnum size condoms, but they were too big for him. We actually nicknamed him "Trojan Man" and would sing the jingle from the commercial whenever we referenced him.

"So I'm thinking you have strong feelings for this guy?" Julie states still going through yoga poses.

"Yes, but he is a bit too possessive of me. He was upset I was on a blind date, and sent me a text early this morning asking how my date was."

"Wait, doesn't he have a girlfriend?" Julie inquires coming out of a pose and sitting on the floor with a serious face.

"Yeah, that's the crazy thing, they've been dating for several years."

"Hmph." Julie raises an eyebrow. She is going over scenarios in her mind. "Well it is not like you're not a good catch. However, he's being a bit hypocritical, no A LOT hypocritical."

"I know. I hope to talk about it with him this weekend. If we can't get through this it doesn't make sense to continue the relationship. Amazing sex and all."

Julie's phone goes off with a version of "Don't Cha" by the Pussycat Dolls indicating a text or phone call from Rob, his choice in a ring tone. He programmed our phones himself. Mine goes off ten seconds later with the same ring tone which means it must be a text.

Hello my lovelies! Let's go out to dinner. My treat. I'll pick you up.

We decide on 7:00. That should give me enough time to make sure my kids are fed. Julie decides to bike ride home, since she did not get a proper workout in for the day, and I return to my office to work.

Chapter 21

I am ready at 6:45. Rob also is very punctual and arrives at 7:00 on the dot. He pulls up to my house and I yell to the kids that I'm leaving, and walk out the door.

"You look fabulous! You're glowing. Did you have sex, and you're not telling me? You did! I'll save you. Say nothing until Julie gets in the car. I don't want you to have to repeat yourself. This way you can think of all the juicy tidbits you're going to share."

Rob puts on a top 40 radio station. "I must do some research so my niece and nephew think I'm cool."

"You're taking them to the NBA All Star game, flying what business or first class?"

"First class for them of course!" Rob states.

"Yeah, I don't think you'll be losing any cool points with them any time soon. Are you sure I can't give you any…"

"If you even think about saying you'll give me money, you're walking." Rob interrupts. Not that he would really make me walk, but I drop the subject. His own sister unfortunately does not allow him to take his nieces and nephews on trips. It is a very sensitive subject for him. Her homophobia is my gain. I do try to reel him in with the spending, I have at least convinced him they don't need to stay in a 5 Star hotel.

I switch stations and I hear the Biggie Smalls and Tupac freestyle. "You want some extra points, learn the words to this."

"Excellent! Record it on my phone please, while I'm driving."

By the time we get to Julie's house, I have played it back twice on his phone, and he has memorized 90% of the song.

"This is my favorite kick boxing song." Julie states. "I used to have seven mack 11's, WHAT? A girl can't rap?" Julie exclaims as she notices Rob and I have started laughing in the front of the car.

"No it is not that." I respond. "We're laughing because you probably do have that arsenal in your house."

"Oh. Hey where are we going to eat?" Julie quickly changes the subject. Sometimes we wonder if she changes the subject to hide the truth, or just to keep us in suspense.

"Tonight is Indian. It is a new restaurant that opened up. I figured we could get to a table first before we talk about Mandy's glow." Rob states. Julie giggles and I roll my eyes and stick my tongue out at him.

The inside of the restaurant is gorgeous. There are individual cabanas and the bright colored saris add to the ambiance. We are seated in a large cabana and before the curtains are drawn, Rob puts in drink and appetizer orders. Julie and I don't object. Usually when one of us orders for the rest it means someone has a secret to divulge, or we were going to grill someone about something. I know Julie is not seeing anyone, and Rob sent us a text he broke up with the Republican so I mentally prepare myself for the grilling.

"Ok sister! So what's going on with this glow of yours! Spill the beans, Julie do you know about this already?"

"Yes, I saw the glow earlier." Julie states.

"It was Michael…" I start.

"The pysch guy?" Rob questions.

"Yes. The counselor. It was amazing, no beyond amazing. We went through two boxes of Trojan magnums in two nights."

"Clutch the pearls." Rob exclaims.

Julie and I laugh. "You can be such a queen, sometimes! It just comes out of nowhere! I don't know why you suppress it." Julie teases.

"I sense a comma, a however, and a semicolon." Rob begins.

I get a slight reprieve as the waitress delivers our drinks and appetizers and takes our dinner order. Before she leaves, Rob orders another round of drinks. We sample some of everything and then all eyes are on me. Without them having to say anything, I know I have to continue my story.

"Well you know he has a girlfriend, but he doesn't want me dating other people. While he was in my bed, he heard a message from Amy wanting to set me up on a blind date."

"What a hypocritical asshole!" Rob expresses. "Next!"

"Well, he has been prescreened. I don't want to give up on him just yet. I plan on speaking to him this weekend. If we can't work it out, then I'll drop him."

"So do we even bother giving him a nickname now?" Rob

asks.

"Let's wait until after her talk." Julie suggests. "Wow he could be the first guy ever that doesn't even get a nickname. So, Rob what happened with you and Confused Conservative?"

"Uh yeah, he splashed holy water on me after we had sex. Each and every time." I unfortunately was drinking at the time and had spit my drink.

Rob handed me his napkin and said "Clean up, aisle six please. Yeah, I could've handled a cigarette after sex. Hell! I could've even handled making a bacon, egg, cheese and pickle sandwich, or whatever food thing he required. The holy water was a bit much."

"Oh come on! I wore a hijab when I was dating the Pakistani guy!" Julie teases.

"Okay Ms. Thing! You were visiting his family in Pakistan, and it was out of respect to him and his family. You dumped him once he pressured you to wear it here."

"And to think I was willing to give up bacon for that guy! Never again will I alter my diet for a man!" We all erupt into laughter. At that point our food arrives. The food is astounding so there is a lull in the conversation.

"So what is going on at this NBA All Star game?" Julie asks.

"I have it all mapped out." Rob pulls out his phone and goes over the schedule with Julie. You would think they were the parents and not me. I'm never worried about my children when they are being chaperoned by Rob and Julie.

The waitress returns and we order dessert. The conversation starts again when Rob tells us his career plans. "Yeah, so I'm thinking I need to take a break for a tad bit. Just spend time for me.

Possibly starting my own agency."

"Excellent news!" Julie and I state at the same time. "You should totally do it."

"Yeah, but I have to time it right. I'll need my bonus to live off of until I'm set. I also don't want to burn any bridges. I do have a huge favor to ask. I've mapped everything out of what I need to do, costs, who I could sign and so on. Could you two go over it for me and see if I'm missing anything?"

"Not a problem! Without question!" We respond.

We finish our dessert and Rob asks for and pays the bill. The car ride home included another rendition of the Biggie Smalls Tupac freestyle. Rob has mastered the song, and even does it without the music. We drop Julie off and pull up to my house shortly after. "Thanks again honey for letting me take David and Sandra."

"Are you kidding? Thanks for spoiling my kids! I know they are in good hands!"

I kiss him on the cheek and head into the house. The house is quiet, so I decide to check on David and Sandra and I see they are fast asleep. I take my Blackberry out my bag. It flashes red, indicating I have messages. Oops! I had not realized I had it on silent. Not too concerned, if there was an emergency, my family would've known to call Rob or Julie's cell. Ah it was Michael and there are several messages.

Michael: I haven't heard from you in a while. Is everything okay?

Michael: Are you mad at me?

Michael: I hope you are okay!

Michael: Where are you?

I should respond. Why didn't he call if he was concerned? Oh wait, he did, I notice on my call logs he called but didn't leave a message. Let me text him.

Me: Hi Michael. I was out with friends. Sorry, I didn't realize my phone was on silent. I am upset with you. Upset that you're not here with me now.

That should hopefully put his mind at rest, and it was true. Although we have to have a major talk, I do miss him.

My phone vibrates immediately. I check the phone to see it is Michael.

Michael: I miss you too! Would you mind if we spend the weekend at my apartment? I want to cook for you and spoil you here.

What woman could turn that down?

Me: I'm looking forward to it.

I take a quick shower then head to bed.

Chapter 22

The weekend finally arrives. Just thinking about what we were going to do to each other was torturous for me. It made the days drag. I did send a few "sexts" and even got some back. I received several deliveries on Thursday of flowers, chocolates, even a singing telegram. I also surprised him and sent him flowers to his office. I have to admit to myself that I am falling for him. I truly have deep feelings that are beyond the physical.

The plan was to arrive at Michael's after I dropped my kids and Rob off at the airport. I told Rob to call me on my cell phone as I would probably be at Julie's. He just gave me a wink letting me know he knew where I was really heading. After I drop them off at the airport, I calm down a bit. Not that I was worried about them with Rob, I have a secret fear of flying. It was a six hour plane ride, I hope Michael and I were not entangled, or I would have to break the mood to answer my phone, I giggled at the thought.

I head over to Michael's apartment. "Oh man! No rain coat?" He greets me while pulling me in for a kiss.

"Since it is the middle of the day, I didn't want to be arrested for being a pervert."

"You can always be my pervert." Michael laughs. "I made you dinner. Come!" He says leading me to the kitchen. We start with a salad, so I thought that would be the best time to start the "jealousy conversation."

"Could we talk about something?" I question him.

"Sure!" He answers, seeming concerned. "What's up?"

"Well I think we need to discuss my dating other people. As I've stated before I have family and friends who feel I should be with someone, and not spend the rest of my life alone. I mean I am technically not alone right now, but the kids will be out the house soon. And you have to admit it is a bit hypocritical that you don't want me seeing other people when you're in a relationship. I of course would be open and honest with you about any relationship I have with someone as I hope you would be with me. Of course if you want to end what we have right now, I would totally understand and respect your decision." I mentally kick myself for the last comment. I really hope that is not what he is going to do.

Michael nods his head. "I had a feeling this was coming. You're absolutely right. I am being hypocritical. I'll be honest. I don't like the idea of you dating other guys. I get insanely jealous by it. I guess you just handle the jealousy better than I do? Or maybe I shouldn't assume much."

"No." I sigh. "It is difficult for me as well, but I realize I'm being a hypocrite to tell you to leave her. If that is what will happen, I feel that has to purely be your decision."

"Well that is a relief. I was worried you were going to end things. I wouldn't be happy if you did. You make my life exciting. I would be angry and bitter if we ended things. I do have to be honest with you. I wish and pray every night that you never date another guy again. I know it is pretty selfish of me. The jealousy thing is my

92

issue and I'll work on it, if you're willing to let me try."

"Yes I think you're worth it." I reply as I stand up and walk over to him and give him a soft kiss on the lips. He pulls me in for a deeper kiss, picks me up and carries me to his bedroom. We spend the next two hours in yet another amazing sexual session. I lay in his arms completely blissful, exhausted, satiated, but wide awake. I glance at my watch. Another hour and the plane should have landed. I roll over to face him. "Do you have a wireless router? Do you mind if I access it with my laptop to track my kid's plane?"

"Don't be silly! Of course I don't mind. We never did finish dinner, why don't we go in the kitchen, eat and wait for the plane to land?" He walks to his drawer and hands me one of his fraternity shirts. It looks like a little mini dress on me.

"I feel like I should give you a secret handshake or something." I tease.

He pulls me close to him, I think he's going to give me a kiss and begins some weird handshake that I will never remember. "There! Now you know it. I can't believe I just showed it to you."

"I'll never remember it. Besides, I rather have a secret kiss."

Michael laughs. "It is taking all my strength not to drag you back to bed now. Let's wait until we know the status of the plane AND you speak with Sandra and David."

This guy is amazing! Our arguments are calm and rational. He is considerate, and can hopefully cook! The sex is beyond astonishing. I can't believe my luck. We head to the kitchen where I've left my overnight bag and laptop. I turn on my laptop and turn my computer around to Michael for his password. He turns my laptop back around and tells me his password.

"They should be landing in an hour." I sigh. "I hate flying.

But I'm sure they're having fun in first class."

"First class? I'm impressed." Michael states.

"Yeah, well their Uncle Rob spoils them. I try to reel him in as much as possible, but he enjoys the finer things in life. Wrong wording. He enjoys the finer things that your average working person would never consider buying. He also believes in sharing with his loved ones. I've asked him not to stay in a 5 star hotel, but I'm sure he ignores me. He is not allowed to take his own nieces and nephew on trips, so he overcompensates with mine. Julie is the same way. She has no nieces and nephews of her own. So they get whatever they want from her. Both Julie and Rob are extremely protective of them."

"Tell me more." Michael prods.

"You're not analyzing me are you? I wouldn't be able to handle it. I get it enough from Julie."

"No!" Michael laughs. "I just want to know everything there is to know about you."

I am more than happy to tell him about my kids, Julie and Rob. In fact, he is the first man I have ever dated that has asked such thorough questions about them. I tell him how David is the constant joker. Always teasing, and playing practical jokes. Being the man of the house, he loves to torment Sandra's male friends. Sandra is the voice of reason. Always defending people, and getting her brother to back off people. I tried putting her in dance lessons, but she followed behind her brother and went into sports. I couldn't be disappointed, because I too was a bit of a tomboy. Julie the secret government agent and Rob the high powered sports attorney.

He tells me about his friends. Mostly from his fraternity, but he has grown close to John. He is close to his brother. It is so easy to talk to him. So much so, I hadn't realized that time had passed by so quickly. My phone rings with a version of "Don't Cha" and I knew it was Rob.

"Hi honey! We have landed and we are in our hotel room. I'm calling to give you the number." I can hear my kids shouting excitedly in the background.

"Oh my! We each have our own bathroom too!"

"What did Sandra just say?" I question him.

"Well I thought it was more appropriate if I got us a presidential suite. We each have our own bedrooms, and apparently bathrooms. Before you give me an attitude, I was comped. The GM was a little tipsy when I met him and I did him a business favor, he is a bit of a show-off, so he told me he'd give me any room I wanted when next I visited. He didn't think I'd be coming back and so soon. Let me put the kids on so you can get back to whoever, I mean whatever you're doing."

I was a bit embarrassed by his last comment, but was relieved when it sounded like he had to call my kids back into the room. I should've known better. He would never said anything like that with them around.

They sound like two years olds that were let into Toys R Us by themselves and told to take whatever they wanted. I decide to let them off the hook. I don't keep them on the phone for long. They wanted to explore their suite, and see what else Uncle Rob had it store for them. I hang up the phone, and shake my head.

"They seem to be staying in the presidential suite." I tell Michael.

"Nice! How do I get an Uncle Rob?"

"Me too!" I respond.

We finish dinner and he produces something that is white with sprinkles. "Is that ice cream?" I ask.

"No. It is called barfi. Try it."

Michael placed some in a bowl for me. My mouth exploded with intensity. I couldn't describe it. There was a milk taste, but also ginger.

"This is amazing!" I exclaim.

"Thank you, I'm relieved you like it."

Once we're finished with dessert, I help Michael load the dish washer.

"So Ms. Jones. Do you think your kids will be calling you back?"

"You don't know their Uncle Rob. He has their entire weekend planned down to each second. They'll be meeting famous people. I'm sure he'll even sneak them into a night club or two. Although he exposes them to a lot, he is a super hawk and makes sure they don't do anything stupid. My kids are not thinking about me right now."

"So I can be a caveman and drag you back to my bed? Well not by the hair, I love your hair, and wouldn't want to pull any out."

I let out a very girlish giggle, and say "I thought you'd never ask."

He grabs me by the hand and leads me back to his bedroom. We spend another two hours testing out the springs in his bed.

"Can I ask you something?" He questions.

"Sure!" I respond. "Ask away."

"How do you feel about me?"

Awesome, he asked it first, so I will be honest with him. It is always awkward when a woman asks first. "I will answer, but whatever you say after, I want to be genuine and true. I don't want you to be pressured into anything. Deal?"

"Deal!" He responds.

"Well." I begin. "I've fallen in love with you. I love you."

I know this is always a dreadful moment for women. We tend to be more emotional than men. It is better when they tell us first, we usually get there before them. I look up at him worried, as there is a delay in a response. I see relief in his eyes, and then an enormous smile.

"That's what I wanted to hear. Because I love you too." He states.

"Then stop talking and kiss me." I exclaim.

He lets out a sigh of relief. "Happy to oblige. Thank you for being honest with me, and trusting me. I promise to take extra care of your heart, and never hurt you." He tells me before kissing me.

"No. Thank you." I respond, and pull him in for another kiss.

After another intense love-making session, I gently kiss around his face several times, and see he has a slight puzzled look. "What's wrong?" I ask him.

"Well, I was wondering if I could meet your kids, if that would be alright with you?" He asks.

"Would you really like to meet my kids, and friends?"

"I'd be honored to meet them." I glance at my watch. It is 10:30. I can send a text. "Would you mind if I text Julie and Rob now? They both have crazy schedules, but if I give them a heads up, they will make it work." I send Julie and Rob a quick text message to see if they are available.

"Hell ya!" I receive back from the both of them. Julie mentions something about wanting to lift a fingerprint. Rob confirms he can meet in two weeks and promises to let me tell the kids. I suddenly realize the cards will be stacked against Michael in my favor.

"Would you want to invite anyone?" I ask. "Since you will be facing 4 of my toughest body guards? The guys from the poker game have nothing on these 4!"

"I'm not worried, but I would like to introduce you to my brother if you are comfortable with that."

"I think I can handle it." I respond. "Why don't we also invite John? I'm sure he's chomping at the bit to find out what's going on with us."

Michael laughs. "Done."

We spend the rest of the weekend in blissful, peaceful ecstasy. I am not sure how we manage to pull ourselves apart, but eventually we part ways. Only to know we would be seeing more of each other.

Chapter 23

"Mom?" Are you okay?" I hear David entering my room.

I roll over and realize I feel like absolute crap. What time is it? It is 8:30. What day is it?

"It is the weekend right?" I ask.

"I wish, wow you look really red, let me get the thermometer. SANDY! Mom is sick."

But I'm never sick. I try to sit up in bed, but immediately lie back down. I feel achy and feverish. Sandra arrives with a thermometer and Tylenol. "Wow! You have a 101 degree fever. Do you want one of us to stay home?"

"Of course not! I'm never sick, this will pass."

"David, go text Aunt Julie and Uncle Rob. Tell them Mom seems to have the flu or something."

"Mom, you sweated through your pajamas and sheets. Here, go in the bathroom and change while David and I change your bed before we go to school."

I do as I'm told as I have no energy to protest. While in the bathroom, I peel off my pajamas and wrap a towel around me. I seem to have developed a case of the chills. Probably because I was sweating. I dry myself off with another towel and sit in the tub and close my eyes. The cold porcelain is welcoming against my skin. I'm not sure how long I'm in the bathroom. I open my eyes to see Julie dressing me.

"Hey, when did you get here?" I ask.

"Don't worry about that, let's get you up and in bed. I have toast and oatmeal waiting for you. I'll make you some chicken noodle soup for lunch and dinner." She answers.

She gets me out of the tub, and helps me to my bed. I close my eyes wanting to sleep.

"Uh, no missy, you have to eat first, and drink some fluids. Not going to let you dehydrate yourself." Julie scolds.

She stands by as I eat and drink and once she's satisfied I've eaten enough she leaves the room. I'm not sure how long I sleep. I wake to Rob bringing in a tray of steaming soup and Vitamin Water.

"Hi honey! Do you want me to take you to the doctor?"

"No, stop worrying. I'm never sick. This will pass." I answer.

Rob sits on the edge of my bed and takes my temperature. "Good, it is down to 100. You still look a hot mess. Probably dehydrated." Rob sits on the edge of my bed and forces me to eat. Julie's chicken noodle soup is the best I've ever tasted. "Now, finish this bottle of Vitamin Water for Nurse Nightingmale."

"Nightingmale?" I moan.

"Whatever, just drink it." Once I'm finished drinking. I close my eyes and fall asleep.

I wake and realize I'm in a pool of sweat. I have completely soaked my pajamas. I peel them off and throw them on the floor. I eventually fall back asleep.

I wake to Sandra's voice. "Mom's naked. Go outside." I feel her pull back the sheets. "Her sheets are soaked. Get some more out the closet. I'll get her in the bathroom and we'll flip the bed." I hear her yelling at, I'm not quite sure.

She gets me out of bed and walks me to the bathroom. "I don't want you to catch this." I murmur. She seems to ignore me. She dries me off and wraps me in another towel.

"Here is your cell phone, you might want to answer some text messages." She leaves the bathroom door cracked. "All clear David."

I glance at my phone. There are several messages from Michael.

Me: Hi. I'm sick. Have flu. Probably because I'm missing you.

Michael: I was worried. Do you need anything? Want me to come over?

Me: No, I never get sick. I'll be fine soon I'm sure. Thank you. Miss you. Love you.

Michael: Love you too. Feel better.

Me: Going back to sleep.

I think anyway. Not sure what they have in mind for me. Sandra comes in the bathroom and dresses me. "All clear. Sorry Mom, he insists on carrying you back to bed. Let's just humor him since he's been weight-lifting. Not to worry, I'll be watching the whole time. Uncle Rob is still here too." She takes my cell phone as David enters the bathroom.

David gently picks me up. Fairly easily. When did he become so strong? "I don't want you to catch this either." He places me gently in the bed and Sandra pulls up the covers.

"Let's sit her up so she can eat." Sandra states.

They gently pull me up and not long after, Rob appears. "Nurse Nightingmale with food coming in."

Sandra and David laugh.

"This is why I love you two. You get my sense of humor. Your Mom totally didn't get it earlier. Let's attribute it to her fever. Speaking of, let's take her temperature. Thank God for digital. You two don't remember the rectal ones do you?"

"Ew gross!" Sandra and David say in unison.

"Down to 99." Rob replies. "We're getting there. If it starts to go up, I say we take her to the doctor whether she likes it or not."

They force me to eat soup and drink more Vitamin Water. I eventually fall asleep. I wake in the middle of the night to another sweat soaked pair of pajamas. I peel off my pajamas and head to the bathroom. I towel off and realize the fever is gone. I put on another pair of pajamas and crawl back in bed. I sleep on the side that is not wet.

I wake before Sandra and David and head to the kitchen for more chicken noodle soup. Sandra and David greet me in the kitchen.

"Should you be out of bed?" David asks.

"I'm fine. The fever is gone." I reply.

Sandra produces the digital thermometer and I open my mouth without her asking.

"98.7. She's good. But you should probably still take it easy today."

They make breakfast for themselves and I head back to bed. I send Michael a text.

Me: All better. I'm headed back to bed to sleep some more to make sure.

Michael: Good! Your body heals when you are sleeping. Let me know if you need anything. I love you.

I head back to my bed and close my eyes. Tomorrow I will be at 100% I have two weeks to plan a dinner and "Michael meeting." I will tell the kids about it tomorrow.

Chapter 24

I must have cleaned my house a million times over the next two weeks. I was beyond nervous for the meeting. Julie and Rob come over early to help me cook and get the house ready. I was pleased to have their assistance. The less I have to do, the less I have to worry about, the fewer things could go haywire.

Julie arrives first with huge bouquets of calla lilies and wine. Rob arrives a few minutes later with sparkling vodka and more wine. "I figured if things start to go awry, we can get drunk and blame it on the alcohol."

We busy ourselves in the kitchen making a feast fit for royalty. All the while giggling like high school teenagers. It had been awhile since a potential has made it this far. Julie and Rob were even arguing over what color their bridesmaid dresses will be. They finally agree on something in the green family.

My kids did an amazing job of setting the table. Sandra went on a cruise with her grandparents last year, and took a napkin folding class. The table was Martha Stewart perfect.

The doorbell rings and David being the man of the house

answers. This is the first time I have ever "brought someone home." So I am a bit nervous about David and Sandra's reactions.

"Oh, you must be Mark, I've heard so much about you." I hear David say.

Thank God I warned Michael about David's sense of humor.

"No, that's the other guy. But if I made it here before him, I have no worries." Michael responds.

David leads Michael and his brother into the kitchen, and I see Michael has the hugest bouquet of irises I have ever seen, and two gift bags. He kisses me on the cheek, and gives me a look that sends shivers through my body and awakens my sexual senses as usual. He hands me the irises, and says "This is my brother, Paul. You must be Julie and Rob. I've heard a lot of great things about you."

"Oh we've heard things about you too." Rob responds.

Julie smiles. "Nice to meet you." She gives Michael a handshake that lasts a little too long. Rob gives me a look. I shrug my shoulders. If Julie is collecting DNA samples, so be it.

Michael passes a bag to David who opens it right away to several gift cards. "Thank you, but this will not endear you to me. I will be watching you." David warns Michael.

"I would have it no other way." Michael responds.

Sandra walks through the door rolling her eyes, "You have to forgive my brother - he tends to be a little overprotective." She gives Michael a quick kiss on the cheek and says "Welcome! I'm Sandra. I was just beating him in a PS3 game, so he's looking to take it out on someone. Since they're still cooking, you are welcome to join us. They probably want to pass around some comments about you anyway."

Michael laughs. "Sure, but I do have to warn you, I take no prisoners, PS3 is my game of choice, I beat Paul all the time. Oh this is for you." He passes her the other bag.

Paul laughs. "Ignore him. He's upset because I got the brains and looks in the family."

Michael and Paul follow Sandra and David into the family room.

"I like him, he's charming." Rob comments.

"Hmmm, so are serial killers. I need more time to assess." Julie replies. Rob and I both laugh.

We finish preparing the food and setting it in the dining room. The doorbell rings, and in walks John with a case of beer. He instinctively knows to walk back to the family room. Julie, Rob and I finish cooking not long after John arrives. I walk back to the family room to let "the kids" know we are ready to eat.

"Ok, we're just finishing up a game." All 5 say in unison.

They sit down at the table, and we immediately dig in. Plates are passed around, the conversation is free flowing. We speak freely on politics, sports, religion. It was an amazing conversation. The debates were often intense, but respectful. It reminded me of growing up with my brothers. The feeling was very comfortable.

So comfortable that it seemed no one wanted it to end. Even Julie who I could see was doing a mental psychiatric profile of Michael. David even invited Michael to his final basketball game for the season, which is tomorrow. At 10:30 pm, Michael and his brother decide to leave, breaking up the party. They offer to help clean up, but David tells them not to worry, he will do it. Michael and I exchange heated glances and a quick kiss that promised a future intense sexual session. He tells me he will pick us up to go to

David's game. John decides to leave with them.

Julie and Rob linger behind to help David, and eventually force him to bed since he has a game. I could tell he wanted to be helpful, but he knew they were right. He reluctantly went to his room. There wasn't much to clean as Julie was doing a lot of it as we were cooking.

Before leaving, Julie turns to me and says, "I hope he is the one for you, you deserve happiness. He seems perfect now because everything is easy. I hope he'll be there during the bad times as well. If not, you will always have us."

"Ditto." Rob responds.

I grab them in a group hug. "You guys are the best. You have nothing to worry about he treats me like a goddess. I'm not concerned." I head to my bedroom. I am exhausted and riding on cloud 9 at the same time.

Chapter 25

Michael arrives promptly at 10:30 am. He pulls me into a tight embrace and leaves a trail of kisses from my lips to my ear, and he whispers "never leave me." He then trails his lips back down to my neck and I let out a deep and throaty groan.

"You are killing me." He says as he pulls away. "By the way, I just want to let you know how hard it was for me to pull away from you. I just don't want your kids to think less of me if they see my all over their mother."

"I don't think they would think any less of you; however, you do have a good point. I'm pretty sure they're just relieved to see me happy." I respond. "I think I will go finish breakfast. Are you hungry?" I kiss him before he answers and pull him in closer to me.

"I'm glad I'm the one that makes you happy." He responds. "But it is probably better if we quit now, or risk scaring your kids for life."

"You're probably right." I laugh. "Breakfast is waiting to be prepared. You're welcome to join me in the kitchen."

Michael holds my hand as he follows me into the kitchen. We exchange one last passionate kiss before I start cooking.

"Where are David and Sandra?" He asks.

"If I know them, probably still in bed waiting for me to call them for breakfast, or the smell of bacon to permeate throughout the house. We probably could have snuck off for a quickie." I respond.

"Don't tempt me." He laughs.

As I was finishing the scrambled eggs, my kids appear.

"Good morning." They both grumble in unison.

"Don't mind them." I warn Michael. "Once they get some food in their system, they will be their usual chipper selves."

We all sit down at the kitchen table, and surprisingly, David and Sandra start a conversation. David, Sandra, and Michael eventually begin a playful argument over who was going to be the best NBA team. David and Sandra feeling they have "inside information" after attending the NBA draft. I end the argument with a reminder that we have a game to attend. The argument picks right back up when we are in the car. I stay out of in lost in my own content thoughts. This was all going so smoothly. I could not believe how well everyone was getting along. Once we arrive to the gym, we part ways. David heads to the locker room with the rest of his team. Sandra sees a bunch of her friends, and politely excuses herself. Michael and I find a nice spot in the bleachers.

I happen to glance around and catch Julie and Rob. Julie seems to be examining Michael. I should've known they would not miss David's last game. They are really being ridiculous. They're probably assuming I want space. I chuckle silently. I pull out my phone and send her a text.

Me: It would be a lot easier to scrutinize Michael if you are sitting with us. Don't cha think?

Julie: Agreed! But we wanted to give you your space. You know we weren't going to miss David's last game. We're coming. Scooch over.

Julie and Rob join us. She gives a stern "Good morning Michael, how are you doing today?" That is her I've got my eye on you, don't try any crap tone. I wasn't too worried. That is Julie's tone with everyone new to our group.

Rob or I usually diffuse the tone. "You guys have good seats, I can heckle the other team from here without being noticed." Rob jokes.

They seem to bond over the game. It was a close, intense game. This meant no probing questions from Julie. I am personally not sure who screamed the loudest. However, if I go by Julie's reactions, I caught one or two impressed smiles from her. The game goes into Triple overtime! However, David's team wins! 103-102. We stay in our seats waiting for the gymnasium to empty.

We walk outside to the parking lot, and Michael suggests we grab a couple of pizzas to celebrate.

"I have a something to finish up in the office, so no can do, but have fun!" Rob replies.

Julie glances at us and smiles. "I'd love to, but I have some work to take care of – I might stop by later, much later with dessert." That was her code for saying, you guys bond, I don't want to interfere, but I'll be by later to distract the kids so you can have alone time.

I smile back and give her a thank you nod. She does a graceful pivot turn and heads to her car.

"That's funny." Michael says "I would never peg her for a Volvo. I see her in a bright red sports car. High-performance. Like a Ferrari."

We all laugh. "Actually, she has a Maserati." David jokes. I shake my head and roll my eyes so Michael knows David is kidding.

We call ahead to the kid's favorite local pizzeria, so the food is waiting for us when we arrive. Michael goes in to get the pizzas and we head home. After we were done eating, David asks "are you two going to smush or do you want to watch a movie?" Before I can strangle him, Michael responds.

"Watching a movie works for me. Besides, I'm not sure I even know what smushing means." Michael laughs.

David and Sandra clear off the table and we all head into the family room to watch a comedy. Michael and I sit on the couch, while David and Sandra flop in various positions on the floor. After the movie, we turn on a news channel. Eventually Sandra excuses herself and gives David a death stare before leaving. He eventually picks up on her hint, and leaves the room.

Once the coast is clear Michael and I attack each other and have an intense kissing session.

"I have Ben and …WHOA!" Julie's exclamation brings the kids running back into the family room.

"Aunt Julie are you okay?" David and Sandra ask.

"Uh, yeah, I just have my hands full and I almost slipped and fell."

That's partially believable. Her hands are full, but it would take a lot more for Julie to slip and fall.

I give her a relieved nod and she leaves to get bowls and utensils.

After we have our share of ice cream, Julie announces "Hey! I have three advance screening tickets for Star Trek tonight. Midnight show. Anyone interested in going with me?"

"OH MY GOD! Aunt Julie, that's not coming out for

another 6 months! I'm going!" Sandra exclaims.

David being the smart ass decides to tease. "Mom, why don't you go with them? I can stay and bond with Michael."

He's good, but not as good as Julie.

"Well actually there can only be one person over 18 per group. Rules of the tickets. All three of us have to go or it will be deemed null and void. It is a bit of a drive, so we'll probably be gone for five hours." The last part Julie directs at me.

Once I hear the front door close I grab Michael and pull him close for a kiss. He pulls away from me seeming concerned. "I don't think Julie likes me." Wow! He is really sensitive!

"She just gave us five hours of alone time to ourselves. She likes you plenty. I'm sure she could've used those tickets at any time. You have no need to worry. Unless you want to talk about it for the next five hours."

Michael seems to ponder the idea. "No, I'm good, shall we adjourn to your room?"

"Yes we shall."

We spend the next four hours entangled in my bed. Thirty minutes changing my bed sheets and taking a shower, and then kissing each other like teenagers in the living room.

I think I better go." He sighs. "I'm not sure how much more I can take being near you and not wanting to rip your clothes off and devour you again."

"You're probably right. They should be here any minute." I respond. "When can I see you again?"

"Anytime next weekend." He replies. "This will be the longest week of my life."

He pulls me into a tight embrace and gives me one long, passionate last kiss.

As I close the door after saying good bye, my cell phone buzzes. It is Julie.

Julie: Be there in 20 minutes.

Me: I had extra time?

Julie: I wanted to make sure. Don't want a repeat of what I saw in the family room with the two of you and probably naked. Me and the kids would probably need group therapy for the rest of our lives. LOL! At tea house. I'm about to get in car, stop texting.

I laugh as I head into the family room to watch a movie and wait for them to arrive. My kids come bounding in, still riding on cloud nine. "How was the movie? Aunt Julie went home?"

"Yes, she said she had to get up early in the morning. The movie was awesome!" David answers. "Michael went home?"

"Yes, he doesn't live here you know! I'm heading to bed. I'm wiped."

Chapter 26

I wake up to the most incredible sexual dream about Michael. I reach inside my secret drawer for one of my sex toys, when I notice this weird lump by my pelvic bone. I feel the other side, and see there is one there. That's odd; I wonder if that is a fibroid that Julie speaks about often. My gynecologist's office is open today; I'll stop by his office.

I really need to find a new one. Last time I was there he told me I had a polyp, but not to be concerned, they could fall off. It was my mentioning it in passing to Julie, and her telling me they could be cancerous that made me remove it. She too was looking for a new GYN, but we really haven't had time to find one. I will put that on my list to do, and text her a reminder to do the same after I get this checked. It is early in the morning, I should get up now and go visit him. The one good thing about him is he doesn't require appointments.

As I walk in his office, I am greeted by the other bad thing. His pushy receptionist, aka wife. "You were here 2 months ago. You are not due for another 4 months. We are not going to get paid by the insurance company."

Unbelievable. Is this what it is all about? Getting paid by the insurance company? I really need to find another doctor. Telling me my polyp might fall off was annoying enough, I can't continue to get bad advice and deal with this pushy lady.

"Um, I feel a slight pain, I need to see him. Why don't you let me worry about dealing with the insurance?"

I was a tad bit annoyed that I had to say that in front of the packed waiting room. Really I have been coming here forever and they've never had a problem receiving payment from my insurance or me, so why give me attitude now?

"Oh okay." She replies. "Have a seat."

I pick up a magazine and wait for my name to be called. They need to update their magazine collection. I realize it is an ob/gyn office, but most of the stuff they have is on raising a baby. I glance around and realize I'm one of two women in the office who are not pregnant. Well the other one doesn't look pregnant, but you never know. The assistant finally calls my name and I am relieved to go inside the waiting room.

I walk in, and half listen to the assistant about undressing and where to wrap the paper cover. I relate it to being on an airplane and listening to the instructions from the flight attendants. The first couple of times you pay attention. After, you half listen for anything new, but you pretty much know what to do. I wait patiently for the doctor to come in so I can get this over with and find another one - today I decide.

"What can I do for you today?" He asks as he enters.

Well at least he is more pleasant than his wife.

"Well I feel these two lumps here. I think they're fibroids. I just want to check to make sure."

He begins to press on the lumps. "No, those aren't fibroids. Those are lymph nodes. That's not me. But let me check inside just in case."

I wait patiently for him to insert the metal spreader. "Yeah, I don't see an infection. You should probably go have a blood test done."

HOLY SHIT! A BLOOD TEST? LYMPH NODES? I start to panic. Before I can form the words he interrupts.

"Why is your anus so red? I am going to do a swab, are you having sex again?"

"Yes, but not anal!" Why is he swabbing there, and what the hell does this have to do with sex?

"Ok, if you don't hear from me, in two weeks, go get a blood test. But I don't see anything."

"Ok. See you in a couple of months." NOT! I say silently to myself. I eventually calm myself. He is not giving out much information. Of course! He doesn't know what is wrong. I'm not even going to ask what blood test I need. I'm not concerned. I will ask my new doctor. My new doctor will do everything and know what is wrong and will reassure me.

I leave his office and decide to text Michael.

Me: I think I have to be the luckiest woman alive to have you in my life.

Michael: No I'm the lucky one.

Chapter 27

The next two weeks pass by with amazing sex, cuddling and conversation. I cannot believe how lucky in love I am! Again! I completely forget about my visit to my gynecologist's office until I am on the phone with Julie discussing my last sexual marathon. I see the gynecologist office calling on my caller ID. Probably something stupid to do with the insurance. I ask Julie to hold on, and click over to the doctor's annoying wife's voice.

"Hello Amanda, we received your test results back, you have herpes."

"What!?" I ask in disbelief.

"Yes, the results came back for herpes. Ok?" She whispers.

"Ok." I answer dazed.

I click back over to Julie and pretend to be listening. I have no idea what she was saying. She of course sensed my absentness. I make up some lie that I'm just tired from all the sex. She laughs and ends the conversation. I call the doctor's office back.

"Hi this is Amanda Jones, so I have herpes? Is there

anything I can take? What do I need to do? I'm not sure how this happened."

"What do you mean? No there's nothing for you to do. The doctor would have prescribed medicine if there was any to prescribe. That's it."

"Can I speak to him please?"

"No he's with a patient, and there's really nothing for him to tell you. See you in a few months."

She hangs up. My head is spinning. That's it, but how? I saw Michael's medical history – wait, I didn't see anything! He told me he was fine. He is the only guy who's medical history I never requested to see. How could I be so stupid to blindly trust him? He lied to me! Stop. This makes no sense. I need some concrete answers before I start accusing. He is a standup guy, he wouldn't do that. I immediately, went to the main source to clear up all unanswered questions in the world – Google.

I found a whole lot of nothing. HSV is passed sexually, there is no known cure. There are two types: HSV1 and HSV2. HSV1 usually manifests as cold sores and are found on the mouth, but can be passed to the genitals and HSV2 seems to just be genitally. The first outbreak can be mild. The person may not realize they are infected. The virus is passed by skin to skin contact. Both viruses are basically the same except for their "hiding spot." The viruses cannot be passed from a toilet seat. They are both killed instantly when exposed to oxygen. The virus will lay dormant, and then something can trigger it to manifest on the surface of the skin.

People usually develop flu-like symptoms during initial outbreaks. At this point I panic. I remember how sick I was several weeks prior. I keep searching. Swab tests are the most accurate way for diagnosis; however the sores have to be present. Blood test will tell you what type you have. After a positive swab test, your doctor should recommend a blood test, then possible medications to relieve symptoms. Wouldn't my gynecologist have told me there were sores? He said he saw no infection, but the area around my anus was red. I need to speak with my doctor.

Unfortunately, I could not get my doctor on the phone. He was hiding behind his wife. "The doctor is very busy. I will tell him you called."

What an annoying little bitch! I am too humiliated to go in the office. Especially since she might announce to the entire wait room that I have herpes, when I don't.

I eventually begin to relax. Obviously he and she don't know what they're saying. They should have at least sent me for a blood test, or given me medications to relieve symptoms, which they didn't. So obviously, I don't have herpes. Michael and I had the STD talk. He said he tested negative for everything. Last straw! Let me find another doctor NOW.

Back to Google. Wait! Here is one. He specializes in Internal Medicine. He's written a book on herpes, and just started a second book. Caring individual, caring staff, a lot of people are tested false positive for STD's because doctors are not familiar with the proper lab tests. Yeah, like my doctor obviously. There is also a gynecologist on staff. Lovely! He has flexible hours. I will call now to make an appointment. I call Dr. X and was lucky enough to get an appointment for that afternoon because of a cancellation.

Now I have to mentally prepare myself to have a conversation with Michael. Texting is not going to work for this one. The thought occurs to me not to say anything to him. But we're in a relationship. I need to talk to someone about what happened. Who else to speak to if not him? Or worse, what if he has been dishonest with me all this time? Or even worse, what if I somehow had it, and

I passed it to him? But I have been tested before, so it can't be me. Herpes is not a dormant virus. It does not hide from tests, at least that is what I gathered from my Google research. He must have it and not have told me. I have to stop. I am really upset and I'm accusing him without him being able to defend himself.

So I send him a text.

Me: Hi Michael, I need to speak to you about something in person. It is important. Please let me know when you are available.

He texts me back right away.

Michael: This sounds serious. Concerning us?

Me: Yes. I really cannot go into it via text or on the phone, I have to talk to you in person.

Michael: Does tomorrow at 6:30 p.m. work?

Me: Yes, that's perfect. See you then. Come to my house.

Michael: Ok.

Chapter 28

I take a quick shower and try to clear my head. This is just impossible. He and I have done pretty much everything but anal, I would have seen something. Why would a swab in THAT area show up as positive for herpes? I decide to stop and get a chai latte to calm my nerves before going to the doctor's office.

I arrive to the doctor's office. From the outside, it looks like a house that was built in the year one. It is modestly furnished, and has a clinic feel, but that is fine. I want answers not a neatly decorated office. A receptionist slides back a window pane and asks me if I am a new patient. I say yes, and she hands me insurance forms and asks me to sign my name on the clip board.

The form takes me less than a minute to fill out. Another benefit of being a mother. Medical insurance forms can be done in the blink of an eye. I sit back down and play a game on my phone as I cannot form proper thoughts at this moment. And if I let my mind wander I will start to panic, and accuse Michael.

After which seemed like an eternity, my name is called. I follow a nurse into a room, where she tells me they need the insurance copay up front. Really! This is so pathetic! Why are people mad at the idea of universal health care again? I pay the fee in cash because that is all they accept. Surprise! She doesn't have change. She tells me she will have change when I come out the room. She really is not winning any points with me, so I ask for a receipt now. I then follow the nurse down a narrow flight of stairs. I am led to an examination room and do not have to wait long for Dr. X.

Dr. X walks in the examination room with a folder. He appears young, but seems very warm. I explain to him why I am there. He does a complete examination. He tells me the same information that I found on the internet. He has patients who have had false positives, he also has patients who have herpes and go on to have healthy relationships with their partners. Well technically he's not fully "my" partner. I'm still sharing him. At which point I start to panic. What if she isn't the dumb little Catholic girl he thinks her to be? What if she is onto his game and is sleeping around? After all, she can't be as dumb as he paints her to be. My stomach starts to feel queasy. Dr. X snaps me out of my thoughts by asking me what type of herpes they said I have.

"I don't know he just did a swab test." I answer.

"That's all? No blood test? Do you at least know what type of swab test he did?"

"No clue." I respond.

See! My gynecologist never did a blood test, he has no clue! I don't know why I stayed with him so long. He then pulls out my folder and proceed to ask me a series of sexually related questions and asks when the swab test was done. I answer all his questions, and I see him taking notes. Dr. X tells the nurse to do a blood test and says he will return.

I thank him as he exits the room. The nurse enters with

labels, test tubes and needles. I proceed to make small talk with her and make sure she is comfortable and not stressed. The two groups of people I never mess with are the ones who prepare my food, and the ones who draw blood. Luckily she is patient and gentle.

Dr. X proceeds to do a complete checkup on me. All the way he tries to make jokes. To relax my nerves I'm guessing. He also tells me that having herpes is not the end of the world. Speak for yourself I think. Some people found happy relationships. Blah, blah, blah, you already mentioned that. I don't need a lecture right now.

I explain to him that I am in the process of finding a new gynecologist. He informs me there is one upstairs, and I could see him. Fine. Let's do this while I am here. Get it all over with so I can get back to my life.

I walk back upstairs to the receptionist area. I tell her Dr. X suggests that I see the gynecologist Dr. Y. The receptionist informs me they need another copay before I can see Dr. Y. This is all so annoying. I pay the second copay. Luckily I don't have to sit in the waiting area for Dr. Y. He is available now. It turns out they are related. He also seems to be friendly and warm. I explain everything to him and watch him take notes.

"It's not herpes!" He blurts out.

Of course not dude! I respond silently. I have found my new doctor!

"It's probably HPV!" He exclaims.

WHAT THE HELL!? I didn't ask that out loud. "Excuse me?" Was what I really say.

"Yeah, they sometimes confuse the two. He asks me if I have had the vaccine, and I tell him no. I am not a believer in vaccines when they are first introduced. Finally I'm getting some answers, not that I want HPV, but this makes more sense, I probably have that. I guess?

Dr. Y tells me it is a virus that forms warts. Oh great I think. But I've never seen warts, so it can't be HPV. He tells me they will do the test for HPV, and I can come back in a week for the results. He tells me I should eat more prunes. It will help to keep me healthy. After this nightmare is over, I'll eat all prunes he wants I think to myself.

I leave the office with some answers, but not enough to put my mind completely at ease. Dr. Y will be my new doctor. I'll talk to him about getting the vaccine when I come back for the results. I head home and have a nice glass, well actually three glasses of red wine, and a bubble bath. I manage to drag myself out the tub and to bed. This drama will end positively within two weeks. I can handle it.

Chapter 29

The next day seems to take a year to finally come. My kids were on an overnight school field trip and were not due back until later that evening. That would leave us plenty of time to talk. The sound of the doorbell indicating Michael's arrival causes me to let out a deep sigh. I can do this.

I open the door and Michael is standing there looking as gorgeous as ever. This time he is not so distracting. He has a worried look on his face, but he grabs me in a warm embrace and ends with an intimate and gentle kiss.

"You know, I could not sleep at all last night." He starts. "If you don't mind, can we jump right into what you want to talk to me about?"

"Sure, let's go sit in the living room." I respond.

I grab his hand and lead him into the living room, and we sit on the couch. "Okay, I have a lot to say. Please let me get it all out before you say anything."

So I tell him what happened with my doctor. I am

surprisingly really calm, and there is no note of accusation in my voice. I was somewhat proud of myself because deep down I just wanted to scream, punch, and kick.

He sighs and covers his face. "So you are saying you were clean before and it is a possibility I passed it to you? Are you sure it was not one of your former partners?"

"Positive." I respond "I was always adamant about going and getting tested together before anything happened. We always went to pick up results together and compare notes. I would even get tested after just in case."

He sighs and covers his face. "Ok, I will make an appointment with my doctor to be retested, and we will get through this together. We just need to get answers first. So I am assuming no sex until we find out?"

"Well I really didn't say that. If I'm infected already, then it has already been passed back and forth. It's too late to refrain from anything. But if you are uncomfortable with it, we can stop."

"Let's stop until we know." Michael states.

"Okay." I reply trying to hide the disappointment in my voice.

"Listen, I don't know if I can go to the poker game tomorrow. This just seems to have blindsided me. I think I'm going to skip them. I just don't know if I can sit in them right now."

The poker games! I completely forgot about them. "I understand." I reply. "I found some articles online. I can send them to you, if you want to read them. The gynecologist also informed me that it could be HPV instead of HSV. They often confuse the two."

"Yes, please do that. I will also do my own research." Michael answers dejectedly.

Michael leaves without a hug or a kiss. I guess he is really upset. I hope he is okay. I decide maybe I should send him a text.

Me: Thank you for stopping by today, and for sticking by me. I know this is tough news, but I appreciate you having my back.

Michael: Always.

Well I was hoping for more, since he is a counselor. Some words of encouragement. But I'll take it. This whole process is hurtful, but I am relieved he didn't seem to know he could possibly have herpes. If I saw that reaction I would have been devastated. I just hope he doesn't have some secret serial killer personality where he could be hiding his true personality.

Now I need to tell Julie and Rob. Wait no. This is a personal matter. Number one relationship rule, when you are going through something personal with your partner, don't let other people in. Besides, this will all be proven false in two weeks. Yeah, I can wait. Julie, Rob and I will have a good laugh at this in two weeks, if I decide to tell them at all.

I decide I don't want to sit in the house by myself. At least tomorrow I'll have the poker game.

I send Julie a text.

Me: Do you have any company? I'm lonely and coming over with a bottle of wine. Tell Rob.

Julie: No need. He just texted me the same thing. See you two soon. I'll start cooking something now. He said he will pick you up.

Always the gentleman.

Chapter 30

I open the front door to walk to Rob's car. I get in and he is playing a rap CD. The Biggie Smalls/Tupac song plays as we drive off. I laugh. A laugh I needed. "I see you're a little hooked to this song."

"Well I don't have street cred, so I just have this song which gets me cool points. Will you be my Tupac?"

"Sure!" I laugh.

So we do a Biggie Small/Tupac duet as many times as it takes us to get to Julie's house. By the time we arrive, my mood is much lighter. We enter Julie's house to be greeted by the most heavenly of scents. She seems to be experimenting with food tonight. Rob and I are in luck.

"My loves!" Julie greets us. "Tonight shall be stuffed lobster with garlic sauce followed by a chocolate molten cake."

"Where did this hooch get lobsters?" Rob pretends to whisper to me. "Julie do you have a Star Trek food replicator you are not sharing with us? Perhaps picked up from Area 51?"

Julie and I laugh. "I have my secrets young padawan. Patience. The force grows strong with you. Now open the wine."

"I have news. I have a potential." Julie announces as we sit down to eat.

"That's awesome!" Rob replies.

"Details! We need details. Have you done his psych evaluation yet? What came up?" I tease.

"Well I haven't done the evaluation. I can wait until after the third date. This one came prescreened. From someone I work with. I was initially worried because it seemed as if we were the only two African Americans she knew and that was the only thing we had that was similar."

"Oh my GOD! I hate that!" Rob exclaims. "I get it too! Just because I'm gay, and you know someone gay, does not mean a happy couple we will make. I'm off my soapbox, you may continue now."

"Thank you Rob." Julie continues. "He is a lieutenant in the Police Force. Has a PhD in criminology, no kids, never been married."

"Can you imagine the pillow talk?" I question Rob.

"Baby how do you lift a fingerprint without that person knowing?" Rob teases.

"Oh whatever!" Julie states as she sticks her tongue out at us. "She is supposed to send me a picture of him, tonight as a matter of fact."

"Well what are we waiting for, let's go boot up the computer. The food isn't going anywhere."

Rob and I jump up and race to her computer. We log in and wait for Julie to join us as we forgot to ask her if the picture is going to work or personal email. Julie enters. "It's my personal email crazies." I type in her password and find the email.

I click on the picture and all three of us open our mouths in shock.

"How do I get one of those?" Rob gasps.

The man on the screen is a dead ringer for Morris Chestnut. He has the same good looks and amazing physique. Never had a blind date come in a more attractive package. There were several pictures that seemed to be taken at some sort of martial arts tournament. His martial arts uniform and black belt upped the sexiness factor.

"Are there any pictures of him wrestling with an opponent?" Rob asks wishfully.

Julie and I laugh and roll our eyes.

"So what's the delay? Why haven't you jumped on him?"

"Right now our schedules don't seem to jive. He is also an adjunct professor at the local community college."

"Julie! What are you waiting for?" Rob bellows. "Don't worry about me! I mean I know Amanda has Michael, and she's all happy. I'll still come around to visit."

We all three laugh, and I start to feel a bit guilty. I should tell them what happened today, but I don't want to ruin Julie's night. We force Julie to send Morris Chestnut Junior an email with all her available dates, then we return to the kitchen to finish our meal. We decide to watch a movie. Rob and I eventually fall asleep in her living room. Julie probably just takes a power nap. I wake to the smell of cinnamon, chocolate, and bread. Possibly cinnamon rolls?

Rob is still sleeping. I decide to leave him there. He has been working longer hours this last couple of weeks to make sure everything is settled at the firm before he branches out on his own. Besides, no one can stay asleep long with Julie cooking. She has made chocolate croissants and a quiche for breakfast. "Good morning! I made extra Mandy, if you want to bring some home to my niece and nephew."

"You know they'd never speak to me again if I didn't." I reply.

"Homemade chocolate croissants? Are you kidding me? This is all going to go right to my ass." Rob teases. We sit down at the breakfast table. Julie places a carafe of freshly squeezed orange juice in front of me. Rob and I devour everything quickly and we clean the kitchen, well the little mess Julie made. Once we are done, he drops me off home. We are so stuffed, the car ride is silent on the way home, except of course for his rap CD.

Chapter 31

The next morning, I receive a text from Sandra asking if I can pick them up from school. Their friend's mother is having car trouble. I decide to run to the grocery store to pick up some items for tonight's poker game. It is at John's house. I decide to make lasagna and garlic bread. That should be quick and easy.

I realize I haven't received a text from Michael in some time. I decide to send him a text.

Me: I just want to let you know, I miss you and I love you.

I receive a response from him, 20 minutes later.

Michael: Me too

Me too? Is that it? I decide to cut him some slack. He's probably still emotional after our herpes talk.

I take a quick shower, then drive to the grocery store. The store is amazingly empty. I get everything I need, and run through the self-check line. I have 20 minutes to get to the school and wait for the buses to arrive. I hope the buses are on time. Just in case, I have a cooler in the car for my cheese. I plug in my iPod and listen to some healing affirmations Rob once sent me, but never had a desire to listen to them until now.

The parking lot soon becomes busy with parents, then buses, then students. My mommy duties will be light today as it seems I only have to drop off two students. We arrive home within an half an hour and my kids announce they are heading to bed. I head to the kitchen to make the lasagna and prepare the garlic bread to make later. The house is quiet, so I decide to plug in the iPod. I see what Julie means that it helps you to create. My playlist is helping me to stay focused. Once I put the lasagna in the oven, I happen to notice my Blackberry flashing, indicating a message. I see it is a text from John.

John: What the hell did you do to Michael? Did he give you an incurable STD? And you dumped him?

It feel as if my heart stops. Before I can ask him what he means, I receive another text from John.

John: LOL! Just kidding. We're cancelling poker tonight. He can't make it, and neither can Alvin and Ben. But I know you cooked something so I'm coming over. Out of courtesy I asked Michael if would object if I came over and he gave me attitude. Whatever.

Why would Michael give John an attitude? Did John ask him about giving me an STD? Perhaps that is why Michael was not so responsive earlier. Let me send him a text.

Me: What did you tell John about us?

Michael: I haven't told him anything, why?

Interesting. His response was quick. Like they used to be in the beginning of our relationship.

Me: He just sent me a text asking if you gave me an incurable STD.

Michael: I didn't tell him anything. Why would I tell him that?

Me: I don't know, I just found it odd that he asked me, especially now. Bad joke.

Michael didn't respond. I guess he is angry. But I can't care right now. My kids are home safe from their trip and John is apparently coming over for dinner. I have to focus on that. I'll let Michael cool off a bit.

I send John a text to arrive at 4:00. Which means he will show up at 5:30.

John: AWESOME! I'll bring dessert. Chocolate cheesecake made by yours truly.

Wow! His cooking skills have really improved over the years. Hmmmm. Chocolate cheesecake sounds like a dessert he was making for someone else. I will have to ask.

John arrives as predicted at 5:30. I knew my kids would wake as soon as he arrived He is so high energy, he takes over a house, forget the room. I decide to ask him about the chocolate cheesecake before my kids appear.

"So you made chocolate cheesecake for poker night? Seriously?"

John chuckles. "That's what I'm telling the guys. I'd appreciate it if you kept it our secret. I made it for my special Valentine's Dinner date. She broke up with me via text."

"Via text?" I roll my eyes disgusted. "Seriously is she still in high school?"

"She was 36! Can you freaking believe it? At least I know now before I got too attached."

"Too attached to who John-John?" Sandra is the first to appear. She has been calling him John-John since she has learned to speak. She is the only one allowed to call him that.

"Some horrible woman who almost became your aunt. Thank GOD I saw her true colors."

Sandra chuckled. "Aunt Julie left chocolate cheesecake?"

"No Sandy! I made it, thank you very much."

"Yes, but how does it taste and should we have 911 on speed dial?" David enters the room.

"Aw man! That's cold. Taste it now! Come on everyone!"

John cuts a thin slice of cheesecake and hands us each a piece of it.

"Wooooooooooooow! I stand corrected and I'm not worthy." David bows to John.

"Thank you, thank you. I'll be taking pictures and signing autographs before I leave." John laughs.

We all have a good laugh, sit down to eat lasagna and garlic bread. The conversation revolves around my kids. Their athletic schedule, Sandra's upcoming play. College choices. John doesn't mention Michael around my kids, and I'm relieved.

We help ourselves to more chocolate cheesecake until John announces. "Well family, you must always know when not to overstay your welcome. The night is still young, and there are women out there who have not had the pleasure of meeting me."

We all roll our eyes and John stands. "Come! Group hug for Uncle John." We give him a hug, then David walks him to the door, as Sandra and I clean up. Once done, we bid each other good night and I head to my room for must needed sleep.

Chapter 32

Two week go by rather quickly, due to my kid's athletic schedules, now we're in baseball/softball season and Sandra's play rehearsals. What made the week hard, was Michael's lack of texting. Although I was working on a project the lack of texts from him was a bit distracting. I eventually decide that since I sent him tons of articles on herpes that I had found online, he is probably busy reading them.

I arrive to the doctor's office early. I sign my name at the window and tell them that I am here for test results from both doctors. She writes my name on a pad and tells me to have a seat. I play a game on my phone, distracting my thoughts. They finally call my name. Before I am allowed to see Dr. Y, they ask me for the copay. This is ridiculous I think, but whatever, I need to know if I was misdiagnosed by my old gynecologist. I won't argue this one. I'm happy to pay the money.

I am ushered into an examination room and wait for what seems like an eternity for Dr. Y to arrive. He finally comes in the room and he is beyond chipper. This is good news I think. He tells me I test negative for HPV and high fives me. Come back in 6 months for your regular checkup. Great, but did you not take notes about why I'm here, I think to myself? I told you I was diagnosed with herpes. Alright. I am not in the mood to discuss this with him again. I just can't. I saw him take notes. What was he doing? Was he pretending to take notes, but really writing his grocery shopping list? Or things to do list? He's not going to serve as my gynecologist. I will wait to speak with Dr. X about the blood test, and find another gynecologist. This one is not going to work for me.

I decide to send Michael a text to tell him I tested negative for HPV.

Michael: Great, so you don't have anything?

Now I am slightly aggravated. I am not quite sure why this is so confusing for him.

Me: No, remember the GYN said sometimes they confuse HPV with HSV on tests. So I tested negative for HPV, but positive for HSV with the first gynecologist. I am waiting to see Dr. X to see if HSV shows up in my blood.

Michael: Keep me posted.

Now I'm more annoyed. His "keep me posted" comment was very indifferent and uncaring. I need to just focus on me for now to get through this. I am a little nervous, but Michael assured me he was clean. So I have nothing to worry about right? My former gynecologist has been wrong about things before.

I sit in the office and look around. It was then that I noticed Dr. X's book was nowhere to be seen. Not even an excerpt. Surely he would have his book in the waiting room? No? Not for me to worry, I am going to test negative.

"Amanda Jones." Hearing my name snaps me out of my thoughts. I follow the nurse inside.

"We need your co-pay."

I'm feeling a little bold at this point. "I am just here for test results." I respond.

"Yes, but you are still going to see the doctor, so a co-pay is required." Oh fine, I say to myself. I just want to get my clear results and get the heck out of here. So I hand her my co-pay and follow the nurse downstairs.

Dr. X comes in quickly. "Who said you have herpes! You don't have herpes."

I let out a sigh of relief.

"Oh wait a minute. You had a swab test done. I still do not have a copy of it. When were you diagnosed?"

"Just recently" is what I manage to get out, but I think "what the fuck were you writing down when I was here for the first visit? Where the two of you passing folders back and forth playing hangman?"

"The virus will not show up in your blood for at least 6 weeks."

I can feel the blood draining from my face. This is absolutely ridiculous. So I tell him I will return in a few weeks. I should probably find someone else, but I really do not want to explain my story to someone else all over again.

So I leave his office feeling more confused than ever. If the virus is passed via bodily fluids, why does it take so long to show up in the system? What is in Dr. X's book anyway? Should he have not told me my first visit HSV takes 6 weeks to show up in your blood? Actually why am I worrying? This just proves that I am fine. I don't have it, and I should start testing for something else.

When I get home, I do another Google search and find a site called wrong diagnosis. There are not many disease herpes is confused with. I do not like how that sounds. I shut off the computer. I need to focus on my kids. I need to think about something else.

BZZZZZZZ. I look at my phone. It is Michael. I forgot to text him

Michael: Any news?

Me: None. I have to go back in another few weeks. Too soon for it to show up in my blood.

Michael: Keep me posted.

This is the first time in my life I feel completely alone. I want Michael to be a little more proactive, but how can I ask him? I want to reach out to Julie and Rob, but they will take my side and blame Michael for everything. I know it can sometimes cause problems brining other people into your relationship. Unless of course, you are lucky enough to have Ben and Jerry in your life. I check my freezer and find three pints of ice cream that are more than willing to offer comfort and a shoulder to cry on. My third and fourth BFF's, they know how to keep secrets and help me focus. "Hello coffee heath bar crunch." I say as I grab the container and a spoon. I head to the family room and select a random movie.

Chapter 33

I fall asleep in my recliner. I wake in the wee hours of the morning with an intense pain in my vagina. As if it is on fire. Luckily my laptop was nearby. I do a quick Google image search for herpes. I frown. I grab my compact and go the bathroom to look. I don't see anything. I can't sit comfortably. I do manage to find a comfortable spot in my bed on my side. However the pain returns. I decide this must be some super yeast infection. I unfortunately don't have any yeast infection medications, but I do have organic yogurt. I have heard many women have used that remedy successfully. I spoon some in a paper bowl and walk slowly to my bedroom. I apply the yogurt with a plastic spoon. The coldness of the yogurt calms the burning. I eventually fall asleep for the night.

When I wake in the morning, the pain is still there. So I decide to run to the drugstore to pick up a tube for yeast infections and hope for the best. The itching seems to subside, but I have difficulty sitting down. Today was scheduled to be a "me day," so I decide to stay in bed and watch movies. My kids are spending time with Julie, so I do not have to worry about them.

I try to stay positive, but the burning is pretty intense. I try the organic yogurt again, and then take a Tylenol. I eventually fall asleep. The buzzing of my phone wakes me. It must be a text from Michael. No, not Michael. It is Frank, my stalker.

Frank and I dated for a year; he neglected to tell me he was engaged. Not quite sure what his fiancée was thinking as we were always together. Come to think of it, Michael and I are always together, well we used to always be together. What is she thinking?

Frank likes to call and text me from time to time to let me know how miserable he is and how I should have told him never to marry her. He claims I'm his soul mate blah, blah, blah. Julie has successfully blocked him from my life, but I guess he has a new phone. I must text her this number – wait no need. I decide to return his text.

Me: Now is not a good time. Going through a lot right now just been diagnosed with a form of genital herpes. Waiting for more tests.

I smile a wicked smile when he doesn't return my text. Wow! Had I known years ago, I would have used this line a lot to get of losers. I sigh. The only thing, this is really not something to joke about, especially not this burning sensation that I feel.

I wait an hour, and hear nothing from Frank. So much for being soul mates. I drag myself out of bed to make myself lunch. It has been some time since I have heard from Michael. Slightly depressed, I decide to text him.

Me: Hi! Miss you!

My phone buzzes shortly after, and I smile as I'm sure it is Michael. That is until I hear "Don't Cha" start to play. It is Rob.

Rob: I know Julie has kids. I'm coming over for pizza and pinto grigio so put some clothes on. Be there by 5:00.

Just want I needed to get me out of my funk. I decide to pop another Tylenol. Although Rob and I are extremely close, he doesn't need to know about my flaming vagina.

Rob appears promptly at 5:00. "Maaaaaaaaaaaaaaaaaaaaaaaaaaaaaaaaaaandy, I'm home." He yells.

I walk into the kitchen where Rob is setting out plates and wine glasses.

I walk over to him, and he grabs me in a big bear hug. "Just as I thought. You are all skin and bones. I got some Sicilian slices and various cannoli. There are regular, chocolate covered, chocolate cream, and banana cream. Now you sit down and I'll get everything together."

"You shouldn't have to…"

"Shhhhh, don't tell me what I should and shouldn't do. Now zip it, unless you're eating."

We spend the first few minutes eating in silence. "Oh my god! This pizza is amazing." I say.

"Nothing but the best for you my love!" Rob replies. We eat most of the pizza. Rob decides we should finish the pinot and the cannoli while watching the "boob tube." As we're cleaning off the table, I hear my phone vibrate. I'm sure Michael sent me a text. He's probably worried about me. I see the text is from Michael. He's probably sent several, I start to worry. When I click on the text, I see it is the only one that he has sent all day.

Michael: Miss you too.

That's it?! Well at least it is not Frank.

"Everything okay Mandy?"

"Uh yeah, you promise not to freak out?"

"No, I don't. I'm gay and whenever anyone asks you not to freak out, the situation usually calls for you to freak out. So just go ahead and tell me."

"Frank sent me a text today."

"That asshole! Give me his number, I'll call him back."

"No, it is okay, I told him I was getting a restraining order this time, so he never texted me back." I try to calm Rob.

"Are you sure? I have no qualms about smashing his face in."

"I'm fine, let's go watch a movie."

Since it is just the two of us, we head to my room. We put on our pajamas and crawl in bed.

"Eat and drink as much as you want, don't worry, I'll put everything away. I have a quick brief to work on, do you mind if I work a bit?"

"How can I mind with you spoiling me? Are you trying to seduce me?" I tease.

"No honey, trust me, I would've done it a long time ago of I was. Well there is something I want to talk to you about. Not sure how you are going to take it. The company is giving me a new car as a bonus. I want to give my old one to the kids."

"But.."

"I know, I know, it is older, but I have an extended warranty on it. I'm not going to make any money selling it, and it has low mileage as I walk everywhere. I just figured it would also help free you up now that you have Michael. I was thinking I shouldn't accept it, since I plan on leaving, but I've given them a lot of blood, sweat, and tears, so the car is rightfully mine."

I know I'm in a losing battle. I don't have the energy to argue with him.

"That is a really generous gift. You really do spoil them you know. Thank you for all you do." It is my turn to give him a big bear hug.

I eventually fall asleep and wake to the spell of bacon, and perhaps pumpkin. Rob and I open our eyes at the same time, or was he watching me? Not sure. "Julie." We say at the same time. "She must be dropping off the kids." I finish.

We both stretch and head to the bathroom to brush our teeth. Never think about skipping out on brushing your teeth with Rob around. We head to the kitchen, and find Julie with my kids.

"Morning! I'm making pumpkin pancakes with cinnamon butter AND brown sugar bacon."

"Morning Mom, Uncle Rob." My kids manage to get out while rubbing their stomachs contently. I'm guessing the first batch of pancakes and bacon is gone. Julie dishes out another batch. Rob and I dive in and she sits down to join us.

"Honestly Aunt Julie, when you're done saving the free world, you should open up a restaurant." David says between belches.

"Thanks babe!" Julie responds.

"Sandy! How is the play going? I'm excited to see it next week. Please text me exact times. I don't want to miss it. I might only be able to catch one showing." Rob says.

"Will do Uncle Rob. I'll do it now before going back to sleep."

"Me too!" David exclaims.

"Before you guys go to bed, hold on a second." Rob states. "Julie could you give me a ride home?"

"Of course!" Julie answers.

"Excellent! Sandy and David, how would you like the BMW in the driveway. I mean, I know it is 4 years old, but if you want it, it is yours."

Sandra and David both jump up excited. "Thank you Uncle Rob." They both grab him in a hug at the same time. Rob knows the only way out of the hug is to hand over the keys. The two of them blaze a path out of the house.

Once we hear the front door close, Rob starts in on Frank. "Julie, Code 1! That Frank bastard is calling again."

"That sneaky bastard! He's good, but I'm better. I will get that asshole."

I decide not to argue with them. I'd have to say how I scared Frank off. I just sit silently as they go on about how they can't believe he is still trying to contact me after all these years, he should focus on his wife and child, etc. I just nod my head every now and then so as not to give anything away.

Rob and I clean the table and Julie heads to my office, probably to limit Frank's access to me even further. She returns 10 minutes later.

"Ok babe, I'm off. I'll catch up with you later. Ease your mind about Frank. He won't reach you again. Rob are you ready?"

"Yes my lovely."

I hug and kiss both of them and watch them leave. My kids are still sitting in the car trying out buttons, and the stereo system it appears.

The pain seems to have subsided a bit. I did have trouble sitting at the kitchen table, but knew not to show any signs of it in front of Julie and Rob. I decide to head back to my bed. I take another Tylenol and close my eyes for a nap.

Chapter 34

"Mom? Oh sorry, didn't know you were sleeping. I needed someone to practice lines."

"Not a problem my love. I'm just resting, not really sleeping."

"Oh, I need to give my drama teacher a head count of who is going to be there on what days. I get reserved seats for winning the lead. I rather not hog all the seats, I'd want to share with others. Do you think you, Michael, Aunt Julie, and Uncle Rob will be coming on different days? Oh and what about John John?"

I was tempted to tell her not to worry about Michael. As I haven't heard from him. He's probably going through a lot. I know I'd be. But still, I wouldn't ignore the person who I passed on an incurable STD to. I'd be doing the reverse. I'd call every day to make sure they were okay. Go with them to the doctor's office. Maybe this is just one of those times when men and women are different?

"Give me the dates and I'll text everyone, and we'll have it all sorted out by tomorrow. Now, give me that script so we can practice."

We spend the next two hours rehearsing. Sandra has it down. I am extremely proud of her. She just has to worry about stage fright, but I'm sure her sports playing has prepared her to fight any fright she may have.

I head to the kitchen to make lunch. The burning and pain seem to be gone. I let out a sigh of relief. I decide to send a group text to everyone to see what days they plan on going to the play. There are only three nights. Miraculously, everyone picks a different night. Everyone but Michael.

Michael: Sorry. Can't make it.

I should probably end my relationship with him. If all were "normal" in our relationship, I would. However, putting myself in his shoes, would I be able to sit comfortably around his loved ones, knowing what I did to him? So he gets a pass this time, but we are going to have to talk. Once the test results come back, negative, we will have our talk.

At least with everyone going on a different night, I will not have to explain his absence. That is a huge relief. I don't like hiding things from Julie and Rob. My kids will notice, but they won't ask.

The rest of the week is spent rehearsing with Sandra, making costume adjustments. Running to the store because Julie and Rob insist on getting a "spare costume" just in case something happens to the first one. But the days speed by.

Julie, David and I attend opening night. Julie almost got into an argument with one of the other stage mothers as Julie purchased an enormously huge bouquet of flowers to give Sandra, and you really couldn't see over them if you were seated behind us. I was able to convince Julie to send the flowers backstage. Sandra was amazing.

David, Rob and I attended the second night. Rob seemed to have even a bigger bouquet than Julie, if that was at all possible. David and I not to be embarrassed again convinced Rob to send the flowers back stage before we took our seats. Sandra was amazing again, I saw Rob blot his eyes at the end. The last night was David, John and I. John also had flowers; however he had the kind that is already made up from the supermarket, you just pick up and pay. So his bouquet was manageable. Sandra was even more amazing the third night. John was on his feet whistling and screaming her name.

John is so excited he insists on treating us to dinner. We decide on Thai food. We spend the rest of the evening praising her acting skills and listening to John's crazy dating stories. We are all so proud of her and caught up in her energy, no one asks about Michael, and I forget to text him. I also forget to notice he hasn't been texting me.

In spite of the lack of communication with Michael, it is an amazing way to end the week.

Chapter 35

My "six weeks" are finally up. I go back to the Dr. X for my second round of blood tests. I decide to send Michael a text to remind him. Should I tell him I'm slightly nervous? No, I decide it is best not to mention it. I'll just remind him I'm going for the second round of blood tests.

Michael: Ok. Keep me posted. I receive my blood test results tomorrow. My doctor assures me that I tested negative for HSV2. He didn't do the test for HSV1 because it is no big deal, and you can't pass it to anyone.

What the hell is his doctor saying? I know you should not trust everything you find on the internet, but every item I have found says you CAN pass HSV1 to someone who doesn't have it. Plus Michael was annoyingly rather chipper for someone who possibly just passed on a virus that has no cure. Stop, I tell myself. You are just having a bad day. You are very nervous, and you are taking it out on him. Perhaps his doctor is correct. You want his doctor to be right. I'll send positive thoughts to his doctor.

I can't think about it too much. I have to focus on an upcoming project I have. It is a huge payoff. I plan on putting the money in my kid's college fund. With this money, I will be set if they do not receive scholarships. There will even be some money left over to buy them cars. If they do get scholarships, it will be luxury cars. I get to work on the project.

At least I don't have to worry about distractions from Michael, like I used to. He seems to be pulling away from me. His texts and phone calls are few and far in-between. I sit and laugh at the irony of it. He wanted me to stop dating other people. Now that I have, it seems he doesn't want to be bothered by me. I finish the project by 1:00 pm and head to the doctor's office. I have exact change for my copay.

"What can we do for you today?" Dr. X walks in asking.

Seriously! Is there any doctor that takes notes and reads them anymore? Well, I do know of two specialist I visit that do, so okay, there's those two. But for those that don't, why do you keep us waiting so long? What are you doing beforehand, if not reading notes?

"Well it has been over six weeks, and I would like another blood test."

"Why are you getting another blood test? Oh! You tested positive on a swab. Sure no problem. Let me call the nurse in to draw blood." He says as he glances in my folder.

I want to ask him why he's bothering pretending to be reading my file, but I just want to get this done.

"You can actually call me. You don't have to come in for the results." Dr. X says.

Ok, so I am a little less annoyed with him right now.

"Is there a good time to call?" I ask.

"No, you can call anytime, if I am unavailable, I will call you back that day."

Awesome, I think as I leave his office. I text Michael to tell him. He texts me back to say he will come over next Thursday to wait for the results. I decide to head over to the mall to do some window shopping to clear my head before I journey home.

At the mall, I buy a magazine, and sit to have a frozen yogurt. Out of the corner of my eye, I catch a group of guys "checking me out." I smirk and think to myself, if you only knew, you really don't want me. I give off the "I don't need a man" body language, and eventually they walk away.

I am just really relieved that this week will be full of projects, sports, and other activities with my kids. Oh, and I'm hosting the next poker night, so I have to mentally prepare for that.

Chapter 36

The next day I receive a text from Michael.

Michael: I am just back from the doctor. I tested negative for HSV2.

Yes, I think. We have been through this. We both test negative for HSV2 prior to us getting together. It is not HSV2 I am worried about.

Me: What about HSV1?

I should probably call him, but I just can't speak right now. My nerves are killing me. I feel a huge lump in my throat.

Michael: I tested positive for that. But my doctor assures me not to worry, because you cannot pass that virus. That's why he never tested me.

My whole world freezes. I actually dropped the phone and head starts to spin. I feel completely nauseous.

Michael: Are you still there?

Me: Sorry, I panicked. I'm feeling overwhelmed and a bit nauseous.

Michael: Well since I make you so sick, I will let you go.

Did I upset him?

Me: That's not what I meant. I am not trying to be a drama queen. It has just been nerves from the project I am working on, reading HSV information on the internet, and now the diagnosis from your doctor. I want him to be correct, and everyone else wrong. I'm sorry, we probably should have had this conversation in person. Please don't be upset with me.

Michael: I'm not. I'll let you finish your project. I'll talk to you later.

I wish I could finish my project so easily. I jump in the tub for a quick bubble bath. With candles and jazz music. That will relax me. Oh, can't forget about a tequila shot. After a 20 minute soak, I get out. Another tequila shot, I sit down at my desktop and manage to finish off the project.

That night, I decided to go visit Julie with my kids. We haven't seen each in a week, and it would be what I need to cheer me up. We walk in on her catching up on Dr. Phil episodes. Surprisingly enough it is an episode on cold sores. He shows a cartoon image of two people kissing, and how the cold sore spores "explode" and that is how you can pass a cold sore infection, or HSV1. Maybe I should ask for a tape of this and send it to Michael's doctor. I am relieved as Michael has never had a visible cold sore. My mind is at rest once again. There is however, something else going on with my body. The burning sensation needs an explanation. After a fabulous dinner, we decide to watch a movie. While Julie and I are making popcorn, she pulls me aside and asks if everything is okay.

"Yeah, I've just been under a lot of stress with a project I'm working on." I lie. I know she knows it is a lie, but she doesn't press the subject. Since it was the weekend, we decide to spend the night, and the kids and I drive home after breakfast. I spent the last 16 hours not thinking about HSV or Michael. It was exactly what the "doctor ordered."

Chapter 37

Once home, I retrieve my phone to charge it. I notice Michael has tried to call me several times. That's strange I say to myself. If he cannot reach me, he will usually send a text. I check my voicemail. He did not leave a message. Not leaving a message equates you really do not want to speak to me in my book. Perhaps he realized he is being a jerk and wants to apologize for everything in person. BZZZZZ. Ah, a text message. It is from Michael. Fine, I'll accept a text apology.

Michael: What I am about to tell you might make you a little confused, perhaps annoyed. So anyway Maureen called me today she did her regular pap smear THREE WEEKS AGO and didn't hear anything so she figured it was all ok. The secretary called today and told her she "needed to come in" to do some more tests, didn't say what was wrong or what she had...but that she needed to come in. They told her to come in for more testing, her pap test came back irregular. I just got off the phone with her, she's worried and so am I.

I freeze as I read his message. Could he have passed it to her as well? I'm so confused by all this.

Me: What did they say is wrong?

Michael: They didn't say. I am really worried what if I (we) passed something on to her?"

Did he not read any of the articles I sent him? If she is testing positive for herpes, he would have passed it to her orally. This is getting frustrating. And what does he mean by "we?" I am the one still testing negative! Well negative in the blood test category. He is the one passing on diseases, NOT ME. I count to ten. Breathe. He really is not this insensitive? He is a counselor! But I guess this is a hard time for him. That has to be it.

Me: When was the last time you had oral sex with her? Sorry if that is too personal.

Michael: It has been 4 years.

Me: Okay so it is something else. Could she be pregnant?

Michael: Haaaaaaaaaaaaaaaaaaaa. ROTFL. *Stop, you're killing me.*

Me: What's so funny?

Michael: She's Catholic so our sexual experience is with a condom and pull out I don't ejaculate inside of her even with a condom.

Really with this religious stuff. It is getting on my last damn nerves. Stop picking and choosing what if most convenient for you. It is not about being convenient.

Me: Does cervical cancer run in her family?

Michael: Her mom has fibroids and may have had cervical cancer ... not sure.

Me: Then that's probably what it is. When does she go back to the doctor?

Michael: Wednesday.

Me: Ok, but again, if you have not done oral with her, and you don't have HSV1 genitally, then it is something else. I am going out of town for a couple of days on business. I'll have my computer with me, and I'll log in on Wednesday if you want to chat.

Michael: Thanks.

Me: You're welcome.

I'm really not going out of town, but he has been so distant, and nonchalant, I want to return the favor. Plus I can't believe I just counseled him. I have to be the world's biggest idiot.

He seemed really concerned for her, I would have like to have 1/8 of that concern, maybe it is just jealousy on my part. Am I being super sensitive? I don't really know her, but I would not like to think I passed anything on to her. What am I saying? I have been testing negative on the blood tests, it is not me it's him. I can sleep peacefully knowing I passed nothing on. My phone vibrates again.

Michael: She may have HPV. Have you ever been tested for that?

Me: Yes. Remember? I came back negative.

This text conversation is starting to get really annoying. Not only does it seem like he is pointing the finger at me, but it is blatantly obvious he has not been paying attention to what I've been telling him about my doctor's visits.

Michael: She got the vaccine for it. Did you get the vaccine?

Me: No, I don't believe in vaccines. Especially ones that are so new. When they give you a vaccine, they are actually injected a live virus in you, so that could be why they picked it up in her test.

Michael: This is all just so confusing. I am wiped out, I'm going to bed.

I begin to panic. Could Michael just be a Petri dish of viruses, and he knows? I'm kicking myself. I know better! The few men I have slept with after my marriage, I made a date to go to the free clinic, and get our results together. Why did I not insist the same for him? My trusting him, was just stupid on my part. The frustration and anger settle in. Why isn't he reading the articles I send him? Was he not paying attention when I told him my HPV story?

After this is over and I am in the clear it is probably best that I separate from Michael. He does not seem to do well in situations when I need him the most. What if my kids are out with him and something happens? I will not make any decisions tonight. I will sleep on it and decide in the morning. I need to go to bed myself. Tomorrow is another day.

Chapter 38

I wake up after yet another vivid sexual dream about Michael. Yeah, that is what got me in trouble in the first place. I think I am being too hard on him. If it were me in his position, I would probably feel all types of guilt. How could you not? He probably just shows it in a different way. He told me he loved me and he would always treat my heart with care, and I would not regret falling in love with him. This whole situation is just stressful for him.

I decide to head to the book store to find a new gynecologist. I head over to the health section and page through the books to see if there is anyone who specializes in STD's. Funny, I don't see Dr. X's book anywhere on the shelf. I don't find much on herpes. Only books how to live with it when diagnosed. Nothing about how to prevent it, that's odd. I walk over to the computer to do a search for Dr. X's book. I can't find the book but I do seem to find some sort of chat room thread about him. It is headed by an RN, she doesn't seem to live locally, but she seems knowledgeable.

I see someone complaining that they are having difficulty finding a doctor and how they are a patient of Dr. X and they are not happy. The RN replies, "let me guess, he has a nice website and he has published a book." I know firsthand that written words can be interpreted in many different ways, but I can read the sarcasm in her comments as clear as day. She suggests that the person try visiting a support group and getting references from the other members. I see someone else has replied and they suggest going to a clinic. Clinics have more experience with STD's than regular doctors. I like that idea! I check my watch. I can probably make it to the local clinic and be home in time for dinner. I quickly log off the computer and head to my car.

I find parking outside the clinic and walk inside. I walk over to the receptionist and ask if there are any appointments. She is extremely pleasant and tells me they are booked today, but they can see me in two weeks. That is bad news, but I've waited this long, I'll take the two weeks. I make my appointment, thank her and head home.

As I am preparing dinner for my kids, I receive a text from Michael.

Michael: Are you pulling away from me?

Is he serious? Why would he text this? Why not pick up the phone so we can have an adult conversation.

Me: No, I feel as if you are the one pulling away from me. Could we talk about this in person?

Michael: Sure, can I come over tomorrow? Early?

Me: How is 9:00 am?

Michael: I'll see you then.

Excellent. We really need to clear the air, and I refuse to do that via text. My kids come in and they have plans after dinner, so there isn't much conversation at the dinner table. They eat quickly and then head out. It never bothered me before, but I am feeling somewhat lonely. I could go to Rob or Julie's, or or call one of my brothers. Instead I decide to do a mental game plan on what I want to tell Michael.

I head into the family room. I can't really fall asleep, but instead take little power naps with the TV on. I can't really sleep until I know my kids are home. I know they are together, so they will be safe in that sense, but I still worry. I wake for the 3rd time at 9:45 pm. Their curfew is 10:00 pm. I sit up and pretend to watch a movie. They know to check in with me when they come home. They arrive at 10:00 exactly. I scold them for cutting it close, and we all head to our bedrooms.

I wake slightly disappointed. I was hoping Julie would be here, so I can tell her everything, but I realized I was just being moody and unrealistic. Just as well, Michael is coming over early. She'd probably have him wiped out if she was here and I told her what has been happening. I drag myself out of bed and start breakfast. It is 7:00, and my kids have baseball/softball practice. They eventually appear in sweats at 7:30, eat quickly and head out. Rob's BMW gift seems to have motivated them to arrive on time everywhere.

Michael arrives promptly at 9:00. I am not sure how to react to him. He pulls me in for a hug, then he kisses me. It is a deep, passionate kiss. The kind we used to share. "I've missed you." He says while tracing my lips with his finger. "Can we promise not to have any more miscommunication between us?"

"Yes, I promise, but why did you feel as if I was pulling away from you?"

"Well this whole, us not knowing if I passed something on to you. I guess I would've reacted differently if I was in your shoes. You seem to be really calm about it."

"Actually, I'm not. I guess I just have my kids which help me get through the day, the weeks, the months. Why don't you text me as much?"

"I just figured you wouldn't want me to text you, you would want your space."

"No, that's the last thing I want." I respond.

I incline my head to reach up to kiss him. This time the kiss is much longer and more passionate. He pulls himself away from me quickly. "Where are your kids?"

"They are at baseball/softball practice for the next 4 hours."

Michael picks me up and carries me to my room. We continue kissing and eventually remove each other's close. Once we are completely naked and I can't take anymore, he pulls away. "I don't have any condoms." I let out a groan. I don't have any condoms either. Once he told me about the Trojan magnums, I threw the ones out I had. I reach for my special sex toy drawer and pull out a vibrator. Michael grabs it, turns it on and while kissing me, he plunges it in me.

Something doesn't feel quite right. I grab his hand. "You have it upside down." He pulls it out. "Wait. I have one for men too. I got it for you, a couple of months ago. We can use it at the same time." I pull it out of my drawer and box. We spend the next hour making out and self-masturbating. Like a couple of teenagers. Once we are done, we lay in bed holding each other.

"I don't like you being upset with me." Michael states.

"I feel the same way." I respond.

"I don't want to, but I guess I should probably go, before your kids get home."

I giggle. "Yeah, probably best they don't find us like this. The psychologist bills alone would probably bankrupt me."

Michael kisses me one last time and stands up to put on his clothes. Once he is gone, I jump in the shower and change my sheets. I erase all evidence that Michael was there. I am relieved we are together once more. I think we are anyway.

Chapter 39

The next few days seem almost normal. Michael and I text each other frequently. Not as much as we did in the beginning, but it is a start. I am happy once again. So happy that I forget about Wednesday – Maureen's D-Day. On Wednesday, I did not receive a text from Michael until Wednesday evening. I sent him several texts to see how he was doing, and only received one word replies.

Michael: Good news. Maureen tested negative for HPV.

I felt wicked for an instant because I was actually thinking "who cares?"

Me: what was wrong?

Michael: Nothing. The pap smear was read wrong. Now I just have to get your results and then we can move on and get closure.

Move on and get closure? From what I have been reading, since I tested positive on the swab, and he tested positive, I pretty much have it. Where will the closure be for me? Before I can get aggravated and create an argument. I decide it is probably best I say good night and clear my thoughts. He beats me to the punch. He sends me another text.

Michael: Good night, I'm going to watch the game.

Me: Good night.

How easy it seems for him to continue with his everyday routines. Routines that have become a burden for me. I no longer have an interest in watching TV shows. I drive with my car radio completely off. There was a time when I would blast the latest rap/pop/rock songs, and bop my head to it, but I no longer have the energy for it.

I head to my bedroom and decide to meditate. Julie has always stated that meditation helps her to refocus when she is about to rip someone's head off their shoulders. I sit and inhale deeply and calmly and try to clear my mind of negative thoughts and focus on the positive. I realize I was wrong to not care about Maureen's diagnosis. She is after all an innocent in this situation. I am annoyed by Michaels reaction, and his wanting closure from me, but decide I probably misread it. He meant it in a positive light. I will take it as positive and forgive him. I then turn my thoughts to poker night. I am hosting this weekend, and I have to figure out what to serve. The meditation does seem to calm me down. My land line ringing snaps me out of my meditation. I answer the phone. It is my brother Peter.

"Hi Mandy."

"Hi Petey! How are you doing?"

"Well I'm coming to town for a few days and wanted to know if it was okay to stay with you and the kids."

"No if you have to ask silly." I tease. "When are you arriving?"

"I'll be there Friday. The company pays for a rental car, so I'll get one and drive over."

"See you then. Have a safe flight."

I return to meditating. I am happy and thankful he is coming. It will help distract me and focus my mind even more.

Chapter 40

Poker night. A night I usually look forward to. Today I am a bit apprehensive. Michael is still not going to participate. Will they ask me about Michael's disappearance? I'm dreading that conversation, especially in front of my brother. Two things help me get through the morning. A surprise breakfast by Julie, and the arrival of my brother. I'm hoping his appearance will cease any teasing about Michael. Peter has been in on several games, and it usually does stop the guys from teasing me. In fact, the only one that usually teases me when he is in town, is Peter.

After a fabulous breakfast and reminiscing, Peter helps me to setup. We have everything ready early, so the only thing I have to do is finish cooking. We finish so early that he agrees to let the kids take him for a drive in the car. It feels good to have a male figure in the house again, even if it is only for a couple of days. My kids are going to the movies with friends tonight. They want to attend the midnight screening of Mission Impossible. They seem to know to ask in front of Aunt Julie and Uncle Petey. Four against one is hardly fair. I give in once Julie announces she will be in disguise making sure everyone is safe. Not sure if she is joking, but neither are my kids. I glance in her direction and I pick up nothing in the body language department. She really is good!

Several hours later, the guys all arrive early with various beverages. I give them 20 minutes to themselves to get the male bonding stuff out the way and catch up with Peter. When I finally make my appearance, John greets me first.

"You know Amanda," John begins, "I will never miss a night you host. I never tire of your cooking."

The guys all laugh.

"Really John?" Ben replies. "I don't think you'll miss any event where there's free food."

The rest of the night goes by with no mention of Michael, and I even win a couple of hands. There were moments where I was alone with one or two of the guys, and no mention of Michael. Good. They're keeping out of it. I love the guy code. I wouldn't even know what to say at this point.

Once the game is over, and the guys leave Peter helps me clean and we try to freshen the room. Ben came with cigars and the smell was still in the room. We throw all the cigar evidence in the garbage can outside the house. We empty almost half a can of Febreeze in the room, as we don't want the kids walking into the smell. Peter watches as I throw all the extra garbage in the middle of the table, wrap in up in the disposable table cloth and pick it up and dump it in the garbage can.

"Well big brother! We're all done. And it seems just in time!" We hear a car pull up in my driveway. I peek out the window and see my kids.

"Why did I never think of that? Those disposable table cloths are the best!" Peter really looks amazed.

"Ah dear brother, it is not your fault; you were born with an incomplete chromosome."

He chuckles. "Good point. Hey do you mind if the kids come and visit one weekend?"

"Not a problem, but you have to check with them."

"Already done, just wanted to double check with you."

"Does anyone check with me first anymore with it comes to those two?" I pout.

Peter laughs. "Well they are good kids, so we know going around you initially isn't a bad thing."

He had a point. I also was not overly concerned my kids were going to New Orleans with my single party brother. I knew he would take good care of them. He, like Julie and Rob, were extremely overprotective of them.

The kids enter the house still excited about the movie. There is no mention of cigar smoke, or who won. Not long after they arrive, we all head off to bed. The poker game was a good distraction. I'm glad I didn't cancel. I will keep up with the poker games. It helps me to forget my worries.

The next day, I actually receive a call from Michael, he wants to come over. We are counting down to my blood test results. I tell him my brother Peter is in town and he can come for dinner. He tells me he can't because he already has plans with Maureen. I tell him he can come over on Thursday. Peter will be gone then; and it is a week before my blood tests were due. Rob found a focus group for my kids, he felt it would be a good way for them to make some extra pocket change. Michael and I would have the house all to ourselves.

Chapter 41

Michael comes early, and we cuddle in front of the TV. I feel safe and secure in his arms, and all was right with the world. He starts kissing my neck. I let out a deep and throaty groan. He must have read that as a cue to pick me up and carry me to my bedroom. He begins to undress me, and I follow his lead and do the same to him. Could he finally be "over it?"

He leans over and reaches for my "special draw." Wait, he surely has to have condoms now? I would have felt like a leper if he hadn't at that moment put his fingers inside me. He knows exactly where and when to touch me. "You are really wet." He moans in my ear. He uses a combination of his fingers, my vibrator, and his mouth on my neck and breasts to bring me to a shivering orgasm. I roll over on my side and my entire body quivers. He rolls over behind me and pulls me close to him. He still has an erection.

I roll over to face him, and moved my hand up and down his penis. "I can't leave you like this." I tell him. Before he could answer I push him over onto his back and kissed him, while keeping my hand in the same place. I left his lips and trailed my tongue down his body and replaced my hand with my mouth. He came rather quickly. I was shocked at first, but then I realized he must not be having sex with Maureen either. Something about that thought gave me a deep sense of relief.

We spend the rest of the night wrapped around each other not speaking. When I wake, there was a note on my pillow. "Sorry, I didn't want to wake you, I just wanted to let you know that I love you and I will always be here for you."

I would have preferred he woke me, but when I glance at the clock, I see how late it is. I must have been sound asleep. He also probably wanted to exit thinking my kids might find us. I forgot to tell him they were staying at Rob's.

I have a lot to mull over. Is this relationship going to continue to be a mutual masturbation relationship? I really don't need a man for that. What's the point? I need an equal partner. I begin to wonder yet again, if he's even read the articles I've sent him. If I have the virus, I contracted it from him. I can't pass it back to him. This is very hurtful, but I need to let him go. What hurts most is that I've let him into my home and he has met my kids, Julie and Rob. I completely opened myself up to him. No man I've dated after my husband's death has ever met my kids or friends, as the relationship never progressed that far. I will worry about it more once I have my negative test results.

Chapter 42

Thursday finally arrives. I am nervous as hell, but I need this to be over with soon. I receive a text from Michael early in the morning that he changes he mind. He does not think he can be with me when I get the call from the doctor. It must be the nerves. I'm surprisingly not mad at him, probably because I am no longer shocked by his lack of concern. I call the office. Dr. X is of course busy with patients, so I leave my number for him to call me back.

The phone finally rings, and I see it's the doctor's office. He tells me I test negative for HSV.

"So I'm in the clear?" I ask.

"Well no, you did do a swab test, the swab test was positive."

"So what can I do now?"

"Well, there is another test. It is called the Western Blot test. It picks up everything. The only problem is it is $400 and it is not covered by insurance. You have to wait at least 4 months from time of infection to take the test."

Great this waiting is killing me, but what choice do I have?

"Ok. Thanks. I will call you in a few months to schedule the test."

I send a text to Michael.

Me: Still nothing showing up in my blood. The doctor is suggesting a $400 test. This test would show everything, but I have to wait 4 months from time of infection to take it.

Michael: Okay, keep me posted.

Is this not the part where you say "I am really sorry you are going through this? Let me pay for the test? Or at least half of the amount?" Give me something! I am completely confused how we just spent an intimate moment together, and then we are at this cold, nonchalant point. Especially when you are a counselor and should be sensitive to people's needs.

I sit down and try to figure out when I could have possibly been infected. I decide to throw in a couple of weeks for good measure since medical insurance is not covering it. I see the best time to test is a couple of weeks before my birthday. Perhaps that is a good omen. I also have my test at the clinic. This latest news gives me a huge migraine. I pop two Tylenol and take a nap.

I wake to the smell of garlic, bread, and is that steak? Ooh! And perhaps apple pie? Julie is here. I sit up in bed. My migraine seems to have disappeared. As I walk towards the kitchen I can hear music playing, and laughter. It seems my kids are there with her. And is that the Biggie Smalls/Tupac freestyle? I smile.

I walk into the kitchen. "Hi Mom!" All three say in unison. I return their greeting.

"Smells awesome in here. Can I help with anything?"

"Nope." I'm almost done. We're having filet mignon, garlic bread, string beans, and apple pie for dessert."

We sit down to an enjoyable meal. We take turns talking about each other's day. There is a rumor that David is going to be captain of his baseball team, Sandra will be the only athlete this year to join the math and debate club, and Julie has a date. I decide not to mention I need to pay $400 for a herpes test and have an appointment at the free clinic tomorrow.

I get up from the table several times, once to get a glass of water. Another to see how the apple pie is baking. Each time I return, I notice some tension in the room. I am about to ask what is going on, then I realize. They are planning a surprise birthday party for me. Are they actually going to try and pull the wool over my eyes? I smile as they have tried to fool me before, and I've stopped them. However, this time, I will let them have their fun.

Chapter 43

Clinic day. I arrive with a book to read. I sign in and sit down. Before I start my book, I do a once over of the clinic. The clinic is very clean and professionally setup. I wait two hours for them to call my name, but I am not complaining. I've waited longer in some private practice offices. This is free after all.

I go to another room where a nurse takes my blood pressure and interviews me. She asks me pertinent health questions. When was my last sexual encounter? Oral sex? Anal? My last menstruation, etc.

I am then told to wait in another room until my name is called. It does not take long for them to call my name. I meet the doctor and she goes over the tests she will administer. I ask her about herpes. She informs me that they only test for herpes if someone has been exposed. I explain to her I have been exposed to HSV1. She then proceeds to ask me if I have any sores, to which I reply no. She decides to do a blood test. While doing the blood test she tells me it is very difficult to contract HSV1 genitially. She draws blood and tells me to return in two weeks.

I have new hope. I trust her. I leave feeling confident. I will get a negative result from her, from the Western Blot test, and I will be able to move forward.

I drive home with a new sense of confidence and a positive attitude. I have 4 hours to work and prepare dinner before the kids come home. Rob manages to appear for dinner tonight. I sense even more secret conversations. In fact, I make a point to walk out of the room on several occasions. I secretly laugh at their deception. They are being obvious at trying not to be obvious. I have fun thinking of ways to keep them on their toes. I return to the kitchen to hear David say "really? Do you think so?"

"Absolutely positive."

"Absolutely positive about what?" I ask.

"Oh that Wilt Chamberlain is the number one basketball player of all time."

I look at Rob. He looks impressed with himself for the "save."

I enjoy our cat and mouse game over the next two weeks. It makes me feel extra loved knowing they are enduring my torture to celebrate my birthday. It is finally time to return to the clinic for my results.

I arrive to the clinic early. I sign in and sit. It is not as busy today, so they call my name right away. The same nurse checks my vitals, and I am instructed to the same room. I wait until my name is called. The doctor informs me I test negative for HSV, and I probably just had a yeast infection. She gives me a prescription for medicine. I tell her that I have had yeast infections before and this felt nothing like what I have had. She explains that it is probably just a bad one. She takes the prescription back and gives me one for something stronger.

Do I even bother telling Michael? I am not even really sure at this point. It seems the closer I try to get to him for support, the more he pulls away from me. No, perhaps it is best I wait for the final $400 test. I do decide to send him a text to see how he is doing.

He responds three hours later.

Michael: I'm fine.

It has never taken him this long to respond. I know he has been busy with work and now he is back in graduate school.

Me: Can you come over this weekend? The kids will be gone.

Michael: I gets off of work 10:00 pm on Friday.

Me: That is fine. I will make dinner.

Michael: See you then

I decide to leave it at that. I don't want a discussion via text. I want it all to be in person. I can wait a few days.

Friday finally arrives, and Michael comes over. He greets me with a passionate kiss. I feel somewhat self-assured by the kiss, but it still does not explain his distance. I lead him into the kitchen and he sits at the table as I prepare a plate for him.

"Can I ask you a question? I was going to wait until you finish eating, but it is killing me." I ask

"Go ahead." He says.

"Do you still want to be with me? It feels like you are pulling away again."

"I am only acting differently because I thought you were pulling away from me."

I wrack my brain. I was still doing everything I normally did, I still send text messages, emails.

"Do you hate me?" He asks. "Because of the HSV?"

"No, I don't and can't hate you for that. You told me you didn't know. Why would I hate you? Besides, we still don't know what's wrong with me."

"I just don't know how I would be if the roles were reversed." He responds.

I take his face in both my hands. "I love you too much to hate you for something you did not do to me on purpose. Everything should be fine after this $400 test."

After a few moments, I move away and tell him to finish eating. After he is done, we go in my bedroom, and cuddle while watching TV. A few moments go by and he asks me if I have ever had anal sex.

"No." I respond. "Have you?"

"No, but it's something I've always wanted to try. You never thought about trying it?" He asks.

"Uh, no, not my thing."

"How do you know you won't like it?" He questions.

"Well because I don't walk around all day thinking about putting anything in my ass and getting pleasure from it."

"So I guess you wouldn't want to try it?" He asks.

Is he kidding? No to vaginal sex, but we can try anal? I turn to look at him full on and get ready to rip into him. He must sense it because he quickly cuts me off.

"No worries, just kidding, I'm sorry if I upset you."

I lay back in his arms trying not to explode. It's just bizarre to me that it seems he doesn't want vaginal sex, but he would push the anal envelope? That nagging question returns. Did he read anything I sent him? You can pass herpes via anal sex. I close my eyes and count to ten. He apologized, so I should be an adult and except his apology.

He chuckles and kisses me on my neck and we continue watching TV. I'm left to my thoughts. How will I know if I don't like it? After everything we've been through, would this bring us closer together? Could we then move back to where we were before this whole debacle? No, I decide. He hasn't been that supportive, and I'm not going down that path until he changes his ways.

He stands up and walks towards my bathroom. I hear him running water in the bathtub. He can't be taking a bath now is he? Before I can jump to any conclusions, he opens the door. I can still hear the water running. He slowly walks over to my bed and picks me up.

"Sorry I stressed you."

He carries me into the bathroom while placing gentle kisses on my face. The bathroom is dark except for the warm glow of lit candles. I can smell lavender, my favorite scent emanating from the tub.

"Um, I could use your help here. I want to join you, but I don't think it would be safe if I carried you in since there's bath oil all on the bottom of the tub."

"Oh sorry." I giggle. I slowly undress and I step into the tub and lower myself in. He settles in behind me. We spend the next hour in a peaceful and content silence. We eventually climb out of the tub, towel off and make it back to my bed.

The next morning I wake to the smell of bacon. Is Julie here? I roll over and notice Michael is no longer in my bed. I walk to the kitchen and find him cooking breakfast. I hug him from behind and ask him if he slept well.

"I always sleep well when I am with you. Now sit, I made you breakfast."

Any doubt of his love for me, I erase from my mind. When we were done eating, we return to my room to watch a movie. I know he cannot stay long. He has work today.

We will be much happier once the results come back negative, and they find out what is really wrong with me. It has really put a strain on our relationship. He must be feeling all types of confusion right now. I do not know how he does it. I do not think I would be able to be so calm knowing there's a possibility I had given someone a virus that had no cure.

Chapter 44

Wednesday. Three weeks before my birthday. Most people would probably be mentally preparing themselves for upcoming festivities for their birthday – especially when you know your family is planning a surprise. My brother's constant phone calls to my kids pretty much confirms the deal. I, however, was sitting in a doctor's office spending $400 on a blood test to find out if I have herpes once and for all. I even have exact change for the copay.

I am finally escorted to the examination room and wait for Dr. X to arrive. He comes in and he is not his usual chipper self. He has somewhat of an attitude. I wanted to ask him what the problem was, I was the one spending $400 for a blood test.

"What can I do for you today?" He asks.

"I am here to take the Western Blot test."

"Why are you taking that, if you have two negative blood tests already?"

Really? Why did I bother giving him a medical history. Should I say "read my fucking file!" Probably not wise to agitate anyone in this office since they have to draw blood. "Well, I had the swab test, and it was positive."

"Oh right." He says. "Did you let the office know you were getting this test when you made the appointment?" He responds in an aggravated tone.

"Yes I did." Okay, there will be no pleasantries this visit. That is fine with me. I want this over and done.

He leaves the room to get the nurse I assume, and returns shortly. "I am just going to do the test." He states.

"Okay," I respond. "Oh, also, I have some insurance forms that I need you to sign, I want to submit this to my insurance company."

"No, it is a waste of time." He responds. "You'll never get the money back. They treat herpes as being cosmetic."

I want to yell at him, but he has the needle in my arm, and he is drawing blood. How is herpes cosmetic when my vagina feels like it is on fire? And herpes has been linked to Alzheimer's? And women with herpes have had complications with pregnancies? Cosmetic? As in a boob job? Are you kidding me? This is not something I want for cosmetic reasons. Hell, health insurance paid for my kid's acne treatments. That wasn't cosmetic? Plus my son never complained about acne burning. Dr. X obviously isn't going to do the forms for me. I will ask for a receipt and claim it on my taxes.

"I'll see you in two weeks." He finally says to me. "It takes an extra week as we have to send the blood to Seattle."

I go to the receptionist desk and make my appointment. I also ask for a receipt. I should probably text Michael.

Me: I am done the $400 test. It was not covered by insurance, and he would not fill out the forms so I can't submit it to my insurance company. I will *get the results in two weeks.*

My phone vibrates immediately. Keep me posted I say to myself before I read it.

Michael: Keep me posted.

I should just start texting myself updates. Can I even do that? I'm sure I'd be more supportive. I laugh. I guess he is not going to offer me any money for the test. It is not that I need it, but it is the principle of it. He could at least offer me half. If I ask him for money, will I look like some crazy gold digger?

I arrive home to an empty house, and walk to my family room to read a book. My kids come in shortly after, and we decide to order a pizza.

I welcome the distraction to speak about their softball/baseball practices. Until Sandra starts teasing David about Maria.

"Maria? Who is Maria?"

"Head cheerleader and all around mean girl." Sandra answers while rolling her eyes.

"Well she's really not obnoxious, you just have to get to know her." David debates.

"Yes, but who wants to know her when she gives you a once over before she speaks to you?" Sandra gives her rebuttal.

"How long have you been dating?" I ask.

"Well we're not really dating." David begins.

"And thank God, she's only slept with half the football team." Sandra answers.

I cringe. I asked John and Rob to have the safe sex talk with David several years ago, so I know he knows about safe sex. But safe oral sex?

"You do know I'd rather you two wait until you are much older to start experimenting with sex. But even if it is oral sex, you should still protect yourselves as you can pass diseases via oral sex." I tell them.

It was as if time froze. Both Sandra and David stop eating and glance at me. David breaks the silence with laughter.

"Ok Mom, uh thanks. Maria and I are just friends, and I hope to keep it that way. She's not my type. I don't really want to talk about sex with you and Sandra right now."

"Ewww, I don't want to know about your sex life either." Sandra ejects. "Mom is it okay if I dye my hair purple? For team spirit?"

"Don't be stupid, of course you can't." David scolds.

"Uh who had the bleach blonde Mohawk one season?" I tease.

"Yeah! Good one Mom!" Sandra cheers.

"Yeah, but we looked mean." David responds.

David finally gives in to his baby sister having purple hair. We spend the rest of the meal deciding what shade of purple, and exactly how much of her head she should cover.

After eating, I return to the family room to do some thinking. I decide I'm going to tell Julie and Rob. I exhale as I realize they are going to be livid with me, but I know I will get the support I need from them. I send them a text and tell them to come over for dinner tomorrow so we can do some catching up. I don't receive a response right away, so I take it as a yes.

I decide to continue reading and eventually fall asleep in the recliner. I sense one of my children coming in and placing a blanket over me. They also remove my reading glasses from my face. I don't move. Their care, puts my mind at ease and I eventually fall into a peaceful sleep. One that I haven't had in months.

Chapter 45

I wake to the sound of "Don't Cha" being played on my phone. It takes a moment for me to fully wake and I realize it is not a text, but a phone call. I pick up my phone and see it is 2:30 am in the morning. My heart begins to race.

"Hello?" I manage to say..

"Mandddy? My Mom, she's, I don't, she's in the hospital." Rob stammers. I quickly sit up in the chair.

"Oh honey, I'm sorry, where are you? Are you okay"

"Home, I can't…she had a heart attack."

"Shhhhh, say no more. I'm getting Julie, we're coming to pick you up and take you to see her."

I quickly leave a note on the fridge for my kids and call Julie as I head out the door.

"Mandy?" She answer her phone on the first ring, sounding a bit nervous.

"I'm on my way to pick you up. Rob's mother had a heart attack. I don't know all the details. He couldn't talk. I figure it will be easier in person. We'll take him to the hospital."

"Okay, I'm here." Julie responds. "Wait! I'll come get you. We'll have an easier time in my car."

Not sure what that means exactly. Unless she has some sort of government car. Or maybe she means she is the better driver, which is true. We arrive at Rob's building and pull up to the front.

"Is Mr. Weston coming down?" The doorman greets us. Julie quickly explains the situation to him. He rushes us into the building and tells us he will watch the car. We find Rob in his bedroom. He is sitting on the floor with his knees pulled into his chest and his head resting on his knees. He appears to be in his pajama pants.

Julie and I quickly dress him in silence. Once he is fully clothed, we somehow manage to get him off the floor and into the car. Julie thanks the doorman and reaches in her wallet to leave him a tip.

"That's not necessary Ms. Julie, I just hope all is well with Mr. Weston's mother."

Julie and I thank him. Rob and I get in the back and I embrace him as Julie climbs in the front. "St. Peter's correct?" Julie asks while glancing in the rearview mirror.

"Yes. I love you." Rob answers and gives us a slight smile. "The both of you." He sighs and places his head on my shoulder.

"We love you too honey." Julie and I respond. I tighten my embrace.

He begins to cry. I gently rub the back of his head. Not sure what to say exactly, as I'm not sure his mother's condition. As if on cue, I glance in the rearview mirror and Julie mouths "she's stable." I nob my head. I decide to not say anything. I'm reminded of a similar scene 14 years ago, except I was the one crying over the news of my husband being hit by a drunk driver. We were told he was stable when we left the house, but due to complications, he never woke from his comma and slipped away from me. I plant several kisses on his head and hand him a tissue every now and then.

Julie pulls up to the front. "You two go in. I'll find parking."

Before we enter, I see Rob fixing his clothes. Ahhh! His brother and sister must be here. I wipe his face and give him a sucking candy. He is about to thank me.

"Shhhhhh, save your strength." He smiles and gently places his forehead on top of mine.

"You can do it." Julie says from behind us. Having a friend with a high ranking secret government job sure has its perks. She must have parked right out front.

"You take his right hand, I'll take the left." Julie says as she stretches her neck from side to side. She is preparing for the upcoming battle with Ron's siblings. Rob doesn't say a word as Julie leads us into the elevator.

The doors open on the 8th floor as if on cue, his sister marches towards us with a stern look on her face. "What's this bullshit that you're her health care proxy? Are you fucking kidding me? Like you care what happens to her? You're too busy chasing penises."

"Ah Susan, always the lady, always a pleasure to see you. Your mother signed Rob as a health care proxy years ago. I guess she wanted to make sure the plug wasn't pulled before she was ready to go. She was probably worried about someone wanting to collect insurance money to pay off the second mortgage on their house. Or is it third?"

I'm glad Julie beat me to it. That was far classier than anything I would've come up with, and that last bit Julie threw in seemed to silence Rob's sister for a brief moment. Susan quickly shook off her shock. "You two don't belong here, this is strictly a family affair!" Susan responds.

That was enough to snap Rob out of his daze. "They are family. More family to Mom than you've ever been. Not only am I proxy, but Mom has also signed a paper giving me power of attorney, and letting me decide who can and cannot visit her if hospitalized. If you don't shut up, I'll have you thrown out of here on your ass which has gotten bigger over the years."

Julie and I smile a triumphant smile. One Weston sibling down, one more to go. Susan was an easy one to handle the other was his older brother Ralph Jr. Ralph was also an athlete, but the biggest racist/homophobe you would ever not like to meet.

"Will you two tone it down! This is a hospital. Get over whatever it is. Hello Julie, Amanda."

That was totally unexpected. The guy voted "most likely to never grow up" seems to have grown up. The fact that he even acknowledged Julie and I was astonishing, as he blamed us for his brother being a homosexual.

"Rob, you three can go in and see her."

The three of us walk past Ralph. Susan and I still holding hands with Rob into his mother's room. Julie gives Ralp a "I'm don't trust you, I'll still be watching you" final look.

We walk in the room and see Mrs. Weston hooked up to various tubes and machines. Rob lets out a moan and freezes . Julie gives his hand a quick squeeze then moves toward the bed. "Hi

Mama Weston! It is Julie. I just wanted to stop by to tell you I love you, and I can't wait for you to get out of here, so I can make you some of my famous paella. Mandy and Rob are also here with me."

She holds her hand out for Rob and me. Rob nods his head and we move forward. "Hi Mama Weston. It is Mandy. I love you and you need to fight. It is not your time yet."

Julie finds a chair and places it by the side of the bed. Rob instinctively sits and takes his mother's hand.

"Mama Weston, we are going to leave you and Rob alone for a bit. I'm sure you two have some talking to do."

Rob looks up at us and smiles. Julie and I both kiss him on top of his head and exit the room. We place ourselves directly in front of the doorway, in case Rob needs us. We stand there in silence, listening, waiting. I see Julie look past me and could tell she is giving someone the once over. A tall, attractive, African American woman is walking towards us with what appears to be three cups of coffee in her hand, I assume her to be a candy striper of some sort.

"You two must be Amanda and Julie. I'm Tiffany, Ralph's wife. I got you three some coffee."

"Excuse me?" Julie states. I'm too shocked to respond. I'm sure Julie was shocked for a moment as well; however, she has a quick recovery time.

"Yeah, we married last year. We had been dating for two years. Long story, but Ralph has really changed. I totally hated him when I first met him. I hope to get to know you two and Rob. I've talked about it with Ralph. He has a lot of apologizing to do. I'm hoping my kids won't grow up with just Susan as a family member, she seems a bit angry."

Smart woman I think.

"Children?" Julie asks. Oh! I missed that part. I glance at Tiffany to see she has her hand placed on her stomach.

"Oh yeah, I'm 3 months pregnant. Do you mind if I go in and say hello to Rob?"

"No." We respond in unison, still a tad bit in shock.

"Do you mind holding his coffee? You can't bring it in the room."

I reach out my hand and take the cup. I am about to drink out of one of them, when Julie gently pushes my hand down.

"Don't drink anything, let me test it first."

I'm too tired and still shocked to even argue with her. Julie disappears and returns shortly. "Everything seems to be in order. It is safe now. It appears they met in a Buddhist Temple."

"So you think the temple is responsible for his transformation?" I ask.

"Either that or that girl knows some serious sexual tricks."

Julie is interrupted by the door opening. Tiffany exits and hugs us. "I'm off to find Ralph."

Rob exits a few moments later. "Well that was, uh, interesting? I need to go find a doctor."

"I'll go look." Julie volunteers. I hand Rob the coffee. It is still hot. "From Tiffany." I state.

"Thanks."

Julie returns shortly with a doctor, Ralph, Susan and Tiffany in tow. I see her anxiously scanning Rob's face for a reaction, and he silently nods his head. The doctor makes his way over and shakes everyone's hand. He introduces himself as Dr. Manuel.

"Can we speak in the room?" Rob asks and opens the door and looks at his brother and sister. Susan walks in first and Ralph is about to follow holding Tiffany's hand. Tiffany stops him.

"Honey, I'm feeling a little peaked, do you mind if I go wait in the visitor's lounge?"

A look of concern appears on Ralph's face. Julie, probably impressed with Tiffany sensing they have a lot of healing to do and need to do this somewhat by themselves speaks first.

"Not to worry, we'll go with her and take care of her."

Ralph exhales, relieved. "Thanks Julie."

Chapter 46

Tiffany, Julie and I make our way to the waiting room. I excuse myself to check on my kids. David picks up on the first ring.

"Mom? How's Nana?"

"She's in stable condition sweetie. No updates yet. What do you and Sandra have planned for the day?"

"We just have practice. We cancelled everything else. We want to be with you and Uncle Rob."

"That's great sweetie. You know Nana and Uncle Rob would both insist you go about your ordinary routine, but you two being around him to support him just might be what he needs. I'll send you a text and let you know where we'll be later. His brother and sister are here."

"Okay Mom. Love you. Tell Uncle Rob we love him too."

"I will baby. Thank you." I hang up with David and wonder if I should contact Michael. I rub my temples. Who am I kidding? I doubt he would be very supportive right now. I decide against it. If he texts me, then I'll tell him where I am.

I return to the waiting room and find Julie and Tiffany in an animated conversation. Julie glances in my direction as I enter the room. "Kids okay?"

"Yes, they're fine. They cancelled their plans as they want to give Uncle Rob their support."

"Her kids are the best." Julie states. "And I'm not being biased."

"Yes, well their Uncle Rob and Aunt Julie spoil them." I reply.

Tiffany rubs her hands protectively across her stomach. "You know I was worried about meeting the rest of the family. I met Susan, and well found her to be how Ralph was when I first met him. Very angry. Ralph has changed a lot. The temple has been a good thing for him, I suggested it to Susan, but she just blew me off. She actually told me to call the gay Weston, if I wanted someone else to join my flakey religion. I was insulted, but I was relieved to hear there was a another sibling. I was hoping since he is gay, he would be open-minded towards me and my baby. Ralph hadn't mentioned him previously. I didn't even realize he had a brother. I was upset that his mother and Rob were not invited to the wedding. I'm hoping they can reconnect now."

"Well, yes, Rob is very open-minded. He also loves kids. Susan's kids are missing out on a lot by not allowing Rob to be a part of their lives." I state.

"Yeah, it seems as if their father has a lot to do with their anger. Ralph is just starting to open up about it. I know he passed away, five years ago?"

Julie made a face at me that said "not sure if this chick is trying to get info out of us or is being sincere. I'm not saying anything else."

I nod my head in silent agreement.

"Do you know the baby's gender?" Julie asks trying to change the subject.

"No, not yet. We want to keep it a surprise. Look, I know you two don't know me at all, but would it be okay if I take your contact information? I grew up without a family for the early part of my life. I was eventually lucky enough to be adopted by someone, but she was an only child, so I didn't have cousins or other siblings. Don't get me wrong, I'm very appreciative of all she's done for me, but I want my child to have access to every family member possible, the more love the better. I'm hoping I can turn to you two for help? I won't go too much into it as it is something he has to work out, but Ralph has admitted that he has missed Rob, and he regrets cutting him out of his life."

"Well, they really put Rob through hell and back. It is really a decision that Rob has to make, not us. With all due respect, you were not there in the beginning, and you didn't see and hear the malicious things they said and did to Rob. If Rob wants it, we'll back him, but we won't push him. Besides it doesn't look like Susan wants a reunion." Julie answers.

"Agreed." I second Julie. "However, if their relationship cannot be mended right away, I'm sure Rob would not take it out on your child. Nothing bothers him more than not being able to be with his niece and nephew."

"Fair enough, I understand." Tiffany answers.

Julie gives her a once over. "Here, let me text you our numbers." She takes a little longer on her phone to send numbers. I'm wondering if she is creating a profile on Tiffany. Actually, I don't have to wonder, I'm pretty sure she is, yeah I'd bet money she is.

Ralph enters the room animated. "Good news!" He shouts.

"She's up and stable. If you two would like to go see her Julie and Amanda. Actually that is probably a good idea before Susan and Rob get into it."

Julie and I both stand up and Ralph pulls us into a tight hug and says "Thank you for everything. Words cannot express my gratitude for everything."

Julie and I are at a loss for words. As we make our way in the hall. I see Julie dotting her eyes with a tissue. "Are you crying?" I ask.

"Mind your business!" Julie answers.

"You are my business." We laugh as we lock arms.

We enter the room to see Susan holding her mother's hand with tears in her eyes and Rob standing back. As we enter, she stands says "I'm third shift, so I'll see you in 24 hours." She walks past us and grumbles a good-bye. We do the same. Except Julie's sounded as if she was concerned for her. Probably just to annoy Susan.

"Hey Mama Weston! You gave us a bit of a fright!" Julie says as she and I move towards the bed.

"Hi girls." She replies. Her voice is a little hoarse, probably from the oxygen they have her on. "Sorry to cause a fright."

"No apologies necessary, we're just happy to see you."

"Ralph is taking the first shift. I'm the second. I told him we'd take Tiffany home if that is okay with you Julie." Rob states.

"No worries sweetie. Are we still on for your house Mandy?"

"Oh, uh yes. I have plenty of food. If not, we can always order." I reply. I forgot all about inviting them to my house to tell them about my herpes tests. Mama Weston's heart attack and the possible Weston family reunion has pushed my herpes confession back. My worries seem really insignificant right now.

"I'm coming too!" Mama Weston declares.

"Not this time." I laugh. "But you know whenever you come home, you're invited.

Her door opens and Ralph enters holding Tiffany's hand. "Mom, this is Tiffany, my wife."

A huge welcoming smile appears on Mama Weston's face. "Come closer sweetie, so I can take a look at you and my grandchild you are carrying."

A questioning look appears on Ralph's face.

"Yes Ralphie dear, I've had three kids. I can tell when a woman is pregnant. There is a glow." Julie, Rob and I all kiss her goodbye and leave the room.

Julie tells Tiffany to take her time, we'll wait for her outside.

Tiffany appears twenty minutes later blotting her eyes. "What an awesome woman. It is kinda crazy that I almost didn't get to meet her."

Rob hugs her. No words are exchanged as still in an embrace they begin to walk down the hall and exit the hospital to the car. Julie has found a legitimate spot out front. Julie and I get in the front and Rob helps Tiffany in the back. Julie turns on the radio and the Tupac/Biggie Smalls free style is playing. Rob and Julie instantly start rapping to the song. Tiffany seems to have a slight confused look on her face but then joins in.

"Tiffany, if you would like to come over, you can, there's plenty of food for everyone." I say.

Tiffany beams a million dollar smile. "If I'm not imposing, I'd love that. Let me just text Ralph, he'll be worried if he calls home and I'm not there. He's very overprotective. That's what I get for marrying a police lieutenant."

Hey, I think to myself. Michael is very over-protective of me. Let me text him.

Me: Hi, sorry I haven't called or texted. With Rob, his mom had a heart attack.

My phone buzzes right away. I smile, relieved.

Michael: Sorry to hear that, keep me posted.

Okay maybe that is not such a good sign. I wait for another text. There will be another text, one of support. Unfortunately, it never comes. Whatever, Rob needs me now. I decide to text my kids.

Me: On our way back to house. Please make a salad and put meat loaf and garlic bread in oven. Coming with Rob, Julie, and Ralph's wife.

Sandra responds first.

Sandra: How is Nana? OMG! What! Who would marry Ralph? Why are you brining her here? Does Aunt Julie know?

My kids know the old Ralph. The Ralph that used to be a racist homophobe. I decide to let them be surprised.

Me: C U soon.

Julie eventually pulls in the driveway. We enter the house to the aromatic smell of garlic.

David greets us first. He embraces Rob first, then Julie, then I introduce him to Tiffany. "Nice meeting you". He says. "Did you leave Ralph's wife on the side of the road? Probably a good thing."

Tiffany thankfully laughs to break the tension. "No, I'm Ralph's wife, I'm glad they didn't leave me, I actually have to use the bathroom."

"This way." Rob says as leads her to the bathroom.

Julie and I turn to look at David. "Close your mouth sweetie, you'll let the flies in." Julie tells him.

"But she's Black!" David stammers.

"Yes and you've seen a Black woman before! Helloooo." Julie states while lifting her arms in the air.

"Is this a joke?" David asks. "You're joking right? Where are the cameras?"

"No joke. Apparently Ralph has converted to a Buddhist and met Tiffany at the temple. She's also pregnant."

"Okey dokey." David responds still looking bewildered.

We all three walk towards the dining room. Sandra is setting the table.

Rob and Tiffany enter shortly later. Sandra runs to Rob and pulls him into a huge hug. They don't exchange words, but their body language speaks of the unconditional love and support. So as not to make the same mistake with David. I introduce Tiffany as Ralph's wife.

I smile as I see Sandra's face go from welcoming, to confused, to bewildered, to back to welcoming. She at least handles it with more poise than David.

We spend the rest of the meal laughing about old times and old stories. Sandra announces she pulled out some old photo albums and left them in the family room. She figured we'd want to see them while eating dessert. She made her infamous snicker brownies – Rob's favorite.

We head to the family room and continue the laughter and good times. The pictures seem to make the stories more sidesplitting. After a few hours, it seems Rob has passed out on one of the couches. David covers him with a blanket. We all quietly tiptoe out the room.

"I'll take Tiffany home." Julie volunteers. "Who wants to come with me to get Uncle Rob's car?"

"I'll go!" David says. "Sandra still has homework to do."

Julie and I smile at each other. David probably has work to do as well, but he probably has a ton of questions for Tiffany, and which teenage boy wouldn't want to drive a brand new convertible Porsche 944?

"Uhhhhhhh." I begin.

"Yes I know Mom, I won't speed in Uncle Rob's car. I'll keep the top up too, so I don't get pulled over by the cops because I look too young."

"Not to worry, I'll monitor him from my home." Julie states. I'm still not sure if she can do that; however, I'm glad she announces it each and every time.

"Wait, what, you can do that?" Tiffany questions.

"Aunt Julie is a secret government agent." David answers. "Top clearance, and a trained killer."

We all laugh. "I do work for the government. Don't listen to him Tiffany." Julie playfully punches David in the arm.

"Should I pick up clothes for Uncle Rob?"

"No, he still has some here." I answer.

Tiffany seems confused, but then smiles. "Rob is really lucky to have you all as part of his life. I hope to see you all again soon." We hug and I watch her walk towards the car with David and Julie. David being ever the gentleman opens the door for both her and Julie, then climbs in the back.

"Here Mom, your phone was in the family room. It's buzzing, I didn't want it to wake Uncle Rob. Here is Uncle Rob's. I was going to turn it off too, but figured I'd just give it to you in case the hospital called." Sandra snaps me out of my thoughts.

"Thanks sweetie." I reply. Hoping it is Michael. It's John. I feel a tad bit disappointed.

John: What's going on? I've been trying to reach you all day!

Me: Rob's mother was rushed to the hospital. She had a heart attack.

John: HOLY SHIT! Is she okay? Rob need anything? You and kids need anything?

Actually I do. I was just diagnosed with herpes and the man that gave it to me doesn't care. I need someone to hug me, tell me it's going to be okay and go punch his face in. Also I probably need a good shoulder to cry on. That is what I think. The selfish desire, always rising to the top first.

Me: She's up now. In stable condition. We are all fine. So far, so good. Thnx!

John: I'm here if you need me. Is it ok to send Rob a text?

Maybe I should've slept with John I think sarcastically.

Me: Sure, but he's sleeping right now, so he probably won't respond until much later. Thnx. Luv ya!

I decide to check on Rob. He appears to be comfortable. I sit in the kitchen reading a book and wait for David to return. I soon hear the roar of an engine, and see a bright red flashy car pull into my driveway.

As David enters the kitchen, my phone buzzes. "Aunt Julie." I say. I see a look of bewilderment on David's face. As long as he doesn't look guilty. He's probably wondering if she really was monitoring him.

Julie: Mandy! Did you want to talk about something? Sorry with everything going on, I forgot you wanted us over.

Me: Nope, I'm fine. Perfect timing. David just walked in.

Julie: I know :p

Me: Good night crazy.

Julie: Good night. It takes one to know one!

I decide I need a hot shower to clear my thoughts before going to bed. My shower lasts longer than usual. I come out and check my phone one last time. Still no message from Michael. I throw myself in the bed and close my eyes.

Chapter 47

I open my eyes what the hell is that smell? I walk in the kitchen to find Rob and David. David seems to be making an omelet for Rob. It appears he has put every known meat and vegetable he could find in the pan. It looks purplish green. Rob looks relieved to see me. If he hadn't gone through a rough night, I would've made him eat David's creation.

"Why is that purple?" I ask.

"Beets! Beets are good power foods. My coach wants us to eat more of them. He gave me the recipe."

"Uh, you have to listen to what your coach advises you to eat?" I glance at the omelet. "Who wants pancakes and bacon?"

"You guys don't know what you're missing." David says as he slides the "omelet" out of the pan on to a plate for himself and Rob. He sits down and takes a bite. He makes gaging noises as he spits the omelet out. "I'll take some pancakes and bacon please."

As I'm sliding the bacon out the pan, Sandra enters the kitchen. "I'm starving."

"You're just in time." I say.

"Uncle Rob , what time do you have to be back to the hospital?"

"Not for another two hours or so."

"Can I go with you?" Sandra asks.

"Sure sweetie, but I'm going to be there all day."

"I know. I'm good." Sandra responds.

"Soooooo." David interrupts. "Tiffany, Aunt Tiffany, what do I call her? She seems nice."

"What did she tell you to call her?" I ask.

"She said to call her Tiffany. I like her. She said I was handsome and quite the gentleman. That woman obviously has good taste and class."

We all roll our eyes.

"Uncle Rob! I'm going to dye my hair purple for spirit week." Sandra interrupts.

"And only you can pull it off my love. Are you going to streak it, or cover the whole head?"

"Ooo! I didn't think about streaks! Streaks would be hot."

"Please don't encourage her." David interrupts.

"Uh, excuse me. Who had the mohawk?" Rob asks.

We all start laughing. "What is it you adults say? Do as I say, not as I do!" David responds.

After breakfast David helps me clean up. Rob and Sandra

leave for the hospital. Once we are done, David informs me he is going to head over to the gym for a workout. He's going to meet Julie.

"Don't push it with her, last time you were sore for days." I warn.

"No worries Mom, I am now in excellent shape." He kisses me on the cheek and heads out the door.

I head to my office to do some work. I check my phone. No message from Michael. I pull out my calendar to make sure I'm super busy over the next two weeks. I am. Score! That way I won't be focused on the negative. So I just have to get through these two weeks, get negative test results and Michael and I can get back to where we started. I miss it. Or I can break up with him. Two weeks and I will decide.

I decide not to be a hypocrite. I send Michael a text.

Me: Hi I miss you. I love you.

He doesn't respond right away. I sigh. This is truly depressing. Looks like I will be breaking up with him. Maybe I should see a psychologist? Maybe I could ask Michael for a referral I kid myself. The buzzing of my phone gives me hope. A text from Michael.

Michael: Love you too.

Well, that is the best I've gotten in some time now. I will take it. I head to my office to work on some projects. I worked a good 5 hours until I receive a text from Sandra.

Sandra: Mom get dressed. Uncle Rob got us Indian food. ☺ B there in 15. His sister is still annoying.

Me: K. Am dressed.

David was here, and probably in the bed sore. Julie is a tough workout partner. I knock on his door. "David, Uncle Rob is coming with Indian food if you're hungry. You have 15 minutes."

"Ok, I'm coming. Thanks."

He won't turn down any meal, my son. I head into the dining room and set the table while I wait for them. Sandra and Rob enter the house as I'm done.

"How's your Mom?" I ask.

"She seems to be doing well. I'm wondering if she faked everything to get us all talking again." Rob sighs.

"Well that is a good thing no? Especially with a new niece or nephew on the way?" I counter.

"Yes, I guess, I just don't know if my sister will ever come around."

David appears not too long after, trying not to show his pain.

"Work out with Julie?" Rob teases.

"You should see how Aunt Julie looks!" David replies.

"You gave me a run for my money." Julie announces as she walks through the door. "I have wine and Italian pastries. A nice moscato to go with the Indian."

"I'll take a glass." David states sarcastically.

"Well half a glass." I say. "Since Aunt Julie kicked your butt."

"Me too?" Sandra asks.

"Fine." I say. "You can have his other half."

Julie pours the moscato, and I start to feel the burning sensation again in my vagina. You have got to be kidding me. I think to myself. I excuse myself and run to the bathroom. I tear through the medicine cabinet. Shit! I must be out of cream. I find a bottle of castor oil my mother in-law left for me. It must be 10 years old. She claimed it cures skin conditions. Well herpes is a skin condition. I grab the bottle and some cotton balls. I pour the oil on the cotton and dab in and around my genitals. The burning seems to stop. I return to the dining area hoping I have not been gone too long. There is a tension in the air when I appear. Of course! How could I forget! My birthday party.

I sit and help myself to some chicken tikka and moscato. So far so good with the castor oil application. I will put some more castor oil on before I go to bed.

"So is anyone on my side with this whole purple hair thing?" David asks, still not over his sister's hair choice color.

"No we're not mohawk man!" Rob responds.

"Exactly! She needs to learn from my mistakes." David says.

"Mohawk man, let's just drop it and finish eating. It is a done deal already!" Sandra states.

We spend the rest of the evening joking, and wondering if Sandra should go completely purple, or just streak.

Chapter 48

The two weeks pass by very quickly. My D-day finally arrives. It does not start off on a positive note. Sandra has a bit of a hair disaster. Instead of waiting and getting her hair done professionally, she decides to let her teammates do it, and at our house. Instead of having purple hair, the girls end up with an orange hue.

I text Julie.

Me: Hey Julie. Hair disaster emergency. Do you think you could send Lizzie over?

Julie: Done. I'll get her there in 20 minutes.

My doorbell rings in exactly 15 minutes. It is Lizzie. Julie's hair stylist who could easily pass for a model. She stands at 6'4" and in in incredible shape. She only wears lip gloss and mascara, but looks like she just walked off the cover of Vogue magazine.

She greets me with a hug and a kiss.

"Where is the hair emergency?"

"This way." I say as I lead her into the bathroom.

"It can't be that bad can it? OH MY GOODNESS! Ok, this is going to take some time." She exclaims while eyeing the situation. She walks around the room and examines the scalps of the girls in various states of disarray.

"Okay, I got this. Mom, do you have any milk in case any of these scalps are burning?" Lizzie asks.

"A whole gallon." I respond. "I'll get it, but do you mind if I leave for an hour or two?"

"Don't worry, these girls are in good hands."

As I leave the room, I can hear Lizzie asking questions and doing triage. I grab the milk and head back to the family room when the phone rings. I look at the caller ID and see it is the doctor's office. I run and pick it up. Maybe they are giving me the news over the phone?

"Hello, this is Dr. X's office. We are just calling to let you know that someone accidently wrote you down in the appointment book. The doctor isn't in. The person who wrote it down should have clearly seen it was marked vacation. Do you remember who it was?"

"No I don't remember!" I snap annoyed. "This is really amazing. If I had cancelled on you last minute, you would have charged me wouldn't you?"

"Ma'am, it wasn't me."

The sad thing is, I think it was her. I recognize the voice. "Fine. When can I come in next?"

She gives me an appointment for next week. This is so ridiculous. I decide to send Michael a text, although I am not sure why anymore.

Me: Doctor was not in today. Someone messed up his appointment book. Have to wait another week for the results. I will keep you posted.

That last portion of the text was probably purely evil on my part. But I need to hear something, anything else from him. A few minutes go by before my phone buzzes.

Michael: K

Wow, that's all I'm getting? Now I'm down to one letter? Well I should be here for Sandra and her friends anyway. As my kids say "whatever."

I walk back towards the bathroom and see the girls in different stages of hair design. Some are sitting with conditioner, some with hair dye.

"Change of plans." I announce. "Do you need any help?"

"That would be great." Lizzie exclaims. In another 5 minutes, you can start washing out hair dye in order of where they're sitting. Then put conditioner on them, and then start washing out the conditioner of the girls sitting over here. I'll be done in no time with your help."

Julie appears not too long after I wash the hair dye out of the last girl. She has two bakery boxes full of brownies. The girls, Lizzie and I all dive into the box. Ahhhh, chocolate cures all. I start to wash out the conditioner of the girls and Lizzie styles in no time. As I glance across the room, I see several of the girls are done. They all have different hues of purple hair, but the hues they have compliment their skin tone. Lizzie was doing an amazing job. The braver ones allowed her to cut their hair in a hip short cut. They were beyond ecstatic with the results.

When the last girl was done, Julie pulls out her checkbook.

"Okay Lizzie, what is my damage?"

The girls in the room all pause and seem to have worried looks. Lizzie smiles. "Although normally I charge more for house visits, I actually enjoyed this one. It allowed me to be creative and do whatever I want. Consider it my contribution to the team. I can write this one off." She says with a wink.

The girls all thank her then envelope her in a group hug. Julie and I help Lizzie escape the hug. We then help her gather her items, and walk her to the door.

"Lizzie, I can't begin to thank you enough. You were truly amazing." I state. "I have no idea what those girls would've done without you."

"No thank necessary! I got my start as a hair stylist by doing slumber parties and experimenting on my friends. This kinda reminded me of that."

"I'm going to go too, since everything is under control." Julie responds.

I return to see the girls have ordered pizza. After they finish eating, I take a group photo and one by one they leave.

I begin to work on my next project, and eventually decide to take a nap. When I wake, I see my kids are still home. "Hey beautiful children, will you be gracing my presence tonight?" I ask.

"Yes, tonight we are. We figured you had a busy weekend worrying about Uncle Rob and Nana."

I smile. I am truly lucky to have teenagers who are respectful and who love their mother. My husband would be proud of them.

Chapter 49

A week later I find myself back in Dr. X's office. A day before my birthday. Now I am the one with the attitude as he is late. He eventually comes in. He is back to his usual chipper self.

"My staff told me to see you first, as you were easy since you are just here for results." He states.

I think to myself. What an odd way to deliver blood test results to someone. It must be good news. I let out a sigh of relief.

"Good news! You don't have HSV2!" He says.

I am super relieved. This is over! Wait! He only said HSV2…

"What about HSV1?" I ask trying to control my voice from shaking.

"Well, yes you have HSV1, but that's not as bad as HSV2. Lots of people have HSV1."

Tell that to my vagina I think.

"So that's why my vagina has been itching and burning for so many weeks?" I ask.

"No, you just probably need to drink more water."

"So I can't pass it on to anyone?" I ask, hoping.

"Well no, you can pass it on to someone who doesn't have HSV1, but again. Lots of people have HSV1. People infected with HSV1 usually only have one outbreak ever. So you probably got this from oral sex. You can't pass it on via oral sex, only by intercourse."

"But my partner has never had a cold sore."

"Well the virus can shed, even when not present, but it is possible he does have it genitally and passed it to you as condoms don't protect against herpes. Or if he has had dental work done, that could cause the virus to shed. But again, lots of people have HSV1."

"I didn't have it before all this." I gather my things and leave his office. I should have asked him if he had it. How could he be so nonchalant?

I exit the office and climb in my car. I decide to call Michael. I can't text this. No answer. I leave him a message to ask him to return my call. He finally returns my call - with a text.

Michael: What's up are you having a good day?

Me: No. I just got back from the doctor's office. I have genital herpes.

Michael: So you have HSV2?

Me: No, I have HSV1. I got it from you when we had oral sex. Have you had dental work done this year? The $400 test picked it up because it tests specifically for those antibodies. If it were not for my kids, I would probably drive right over a cliff right now.

Michael: Actually, I have had dental work done. Sorry to make you feel that way, I guess I'll go.

This time I refuse to stop him. Have I been stupid all this time? After my nerves settle I decide to send Michael a text.

Me: I am sorry about the driving over a cliff comment. I don't blame you for anything.

I do not receive a response from him, but I'm no longer surprised and I'm tired of making excuses for him. I shouldn't have even sent that text.

I can't sleep. My mind is still swimming. I decide to send Michael one last text.

Me: I hope I'm not waking you. I just can't sleep right now. I'm confused and crazed. I have answers, but I still have questions. I just want to let you know, I don't blame you for anything. This is just very stressful.

Michael: I know what you mean.

As I finish reading the text. I break down. I finally realize that I was going through this process alone, and will probably continue to go through it alone. The waterworks start flowing, and I eventually cry myself to sleep.

Chapter 50

My cell phone buzzing wakes me. My birthday. A text from Rob. He is always the first to wish me a happy birthday with some graphic picture. This year is a cake with penis candles. He has to always be the first, so he sends a text and he'll give me a call later. I receive tons of text messages, phone calls, emails, facebook messages, one after the other. The land line phone calls start soon.

I had not heard from Michael, I thought it was pretty odd, but he has been working long hours, maybe he is still asleep. He also probably doesn't want to ruin the surprise. I walk into the kitchen to find my kids arguing over making me breakfast. I am relieved it is a weekend, as they have made a complete mess of the kitchen.

"Happy Birthday to the best mom ever!" They shout as they run over to embrace me in a bear hug. When we part, I see there is flour down my shirt.

"Do you two need some help?" I ask.

"No! You just sit down. We have this under control." They respond.

I sit and I watch as they run around the kitchen. Every now and then, they would criticize each other's technique. I'm hoping David got over listening to his coach for beet recipes. A few moments later, a dish is placed in front of me with pumpkin pancakes, Canadian bacon and scrambled eggs. I didn't each much yesterday, so I scarf everything down.

Julie arrives just as I put the last forkful in my mouth. She is carrying a huge bouquet of gerbera daisies, and a bottle of my favorite expensive moscato.

"Happy Birthday honey!" She shouts.

"Thank you, but this is not necessary."

"Yes it is! So listen," She continues. "The kids and I are taking you out to dinner at 5:00, so be ready! I'll be back by 4:30. Love ya!"

"Love ya too!" I respond.

After she leaves, my kids come bounding back in the room with gifts. I can tell Sandra wrapped one and David wrapped the other. Sandra is completely my little clone. A tomboy at heart, but when it comes to "domestic things" we put great care and patience in them. David, just wraps until the box is covered, and places tape strategically around the box. Sandra hands me David's box first.

I unwrap it to find a gorgeous red shirt. "It's beautiful I say. I'll try it on now?"

"Open mine next." Sandra responds. I open hers to find a pair of fitted black pants, with red accessories.

"Are you two worried about my fashion style?" I ask laughing.

"Of course not! You are the hippest mother ever, we just

didn't want you to have to worry about anything today. So this is what you will be wearing."

My eyes start to tear up. "I have to be the luckiest mother in the world!" I say as I gather the two of them in a hug.

"We are going to have a Star Wars marathon today. We will break to make you lunch, then break to go out to dinner."

I make my way into the family room and plop down in the recliner.

Two Star Wars movies later, there was still nothing from Michael. I thought that was very odd. Maybe he is part of the surprise for me? That has to be the reason. My kids run to the kitchen to make lunch. They tell me it will be something light since we are going out later.

At 3:30 we stop our marathon to get ready. David appears wearing a blue shirt, with matching tie. Sandra in a matching blue dress. "You two look amazing!" I gush.

"Yes we do." David responds, ever the confident one. "It is because we come from a pretty strong gene pool."

Julie arrives exactly at 4:30, in a stretch limo. "Everyone ready? I arranged for a car, as I need a drink or two after the day I've had."

She usually does not get frazzled, I send her a "what is wrong face?" She sends me a "no need to worry." In what seems like a few minutes, we arrive at my favorite Italian restaurant. We are ushered to a room where I am surprised by my friends. Rob leads the room in singing happy birthday. I see him and Julie exchange disapproving scowls. I scan the room for Michael. Could he be in the bathroom? Julie pulls me in for a hug, and says "That prick isn't here. We will talk later."

I spend the rest of the evening enjoying everyone's company, but feeling confused. Why would he not be here? Why would he not even call or text me? Tiffany and Ralph are even here! Julie and I finally have a moment alone.

"What the fuck is going on with you two?" She asks while we are in the bathroom.

"I am not sure what you mean." I respond.

"Where is Michael, why isn't he here? He said he would be weeks ago, but gave me some bullshit excuse."

I feel a knot in my stomach. "Well we haven't been seeing much of each other lately, he is back in school, and I have had all the projects to do."

Julie stares at me intensely. "Fine, I will wait for you to tell me. Don't let his absence get you down. The people here tonight care and genuinely love you."

She is right. I have to start living my life again for my children and me. I spend the rest of the night eating, drinking, and enjoying everyone. When it is time to leave, we climb back into the car and head home. Julie gets out with an overnight bag. I also see her car is parked in my driveway. I smile.

"If I am ever on my deathbed, will you be able to tell me what you really do?" I ask her.

"Possibly, but we will have to make sure it is terminal. If they find a cure for what takes you out at the last minute. They will make me kill you, and we'll have to go on the run."

We giggle and hug as we enter my house.

"Thank you for an amazing evening!" I say.

"No thanks necessary honey!" She responds.

Chapter 51

Two days go by and Michael comes over in the morning. He has a bouquet of flowers and a card. He tells me he is sorry for not calling or texting me for my birthday. He just figured I would be busy with everyone and he didn't want to bother me. I am trying to be adult and forgive him. If this were any other time in my life, he would've been out of here. The only reason he is still around is the emotional roller coaster he has put me through. Part of me is also hoping that the "great guy" I've been told and thought he was is going to return.

After telling him my kids aren't here, we fall into our now usual routine of eating, watching a movie, kissing, fondling, him using a vibrator on me, me performing oral sex on him. I cry myself to sleep. He either doesn't notice, or doesn't care. I finally realize, a few days later by text, it is the later.

Michael: I feel I have to tell you everything about my relationship with Maureen. She decided to tell her parents about us, and they want to arrange a meeting.

Me: Ok. Thanks for telling me.

That is really odd. Why would she risk the wrath of her parents to tell her she is dating a non-Catholic I think? Surely their response will be no different the first time she told them about him. I finally have my answer a week later, also via text.

Michael: We met with Maureen's parents, and my parents. We had a long conversation and after everything, we decided we would get married sometime next year. I'm going to convert and become Catholic.

Is he fucking kidding me? I knew he was pulling away from me and didn't care anymore. I also realized that we were going separate ways. I mean you don't miss someone's birthday you truly care about. What I can't believe is that he is actually telling me this via a text message.

Me: Well, this is a nice easy way for you to end things isn't it? I guess you're getting you're happily ever after.

Michael: I am not sure why you are trying to make me look like a bad guy. Does it make this easier? Do you think I've been leading you on?

I am completely and totally infuriated at this point. I am trying to remain calm. After counting to 20, I respond.

Me: I really just thought I was worth more to you than to have heard this news via a text. I guess I was wrong. This is all a little too convenient to have been decided in such a short period of time.

No more apologizes from me. He should be the one with the apologies. Come to think of it. I have not heard one from him. Since this whole herpes mess started. I cannot believe how stupid I was to trust this guy, introduce him to my kids, just hand over my heart. To keep making excuse for him.

Michael: I was hoping we could stay connected and remain friends. You don't have to say anything now. Maybe we can meet in person?

As if there is anything else to say. I turn off my phone and cry myself to sleep. I realize I am not upset at his marrying Maureen, rather at his treatment of me the whole time. It hits me like an atom bomb. Everything was going smoothly until I contracted herpes. He started pulling away from me and the kicker is I contracted it from him. He was never there for me. I went through this by myself. I was so far in love with him, I never realized it. Wow! I was his escape girl. How could I be so stupid? Every time there was a problem with Maureen, was probably when he called me.

I decide to send Julie and Rob a text message.

Me: Michael and I are over. He just informed me he's marrying Maureen and becoming Catholic.

Julie: Loser! I never did trust him fully. Idiot!

Rob: I hope his cock falls off and lands in his ass.

I laugh. Rob always comes up with the best punishments.

Julie and Rob: We knew something was going on. You've put on too much weight. You need company?

Me: I don't care, I'm done with him. I'm fine. Really. Love you.

Julie and Rob: Love you too!

Chapter 52

Two weeks have passed and I've developed a regimen of egg whites with pesto, salads and kickboxing. I have shed 6 pounds. Rob, Julie and my kids seem to know not to mention Michael. It is business as usual. My kids are in New Orleans visiting Peter. Rob's mother is out of the hospital and he has been staying with her. Julie has finally made a date with the Morris Chestnut look alike. In fact, tonight is the date. I know I will have to explain everything to them soon. I'm sure they realized there is more going on than just Michael getting married and converting. I decide to give it another week, until things settle with Rob's mother.

I have a late workout, and as I'm getting out of the shower, I hear my cell phone ring. It is 11:30 pm. I feel a bit concerned by the time with my kids being away. It is Julie, I hope she is okay. Actually I hope her date didn't try anything stupid, or he'd be in the hospital. Maybe she needs bail money.

"Hello?" I answer.

"Hey Mandy, hold on while I click over Rob. I didn't kill anyone, I don't need bail money. Rob already asked."

Julie clicks back over. "Okay, no questions until the end. I know we usually don't do it this way, but there is a reason. So let me tell the story. So Morris Chestnut takes me to that super loud BBQ restaurant with the supersized drinks. Yeah, I know, gross! He's gorgeous though and a great guy. So I'd just have to help him with his restaurant choices, that's no biggie, I can actually live with that. But Amanda, you will never guess who I saw! Michael! That loser was with another woman. What a waste of time. You should have let me run a check on him and spared you."

My heart leaped into my throat. What? I thought he was going to focus on his relationship and marry Maureen? Become Catholic?

"Julie, how do you know it wasn't Maureen?" I ask.

"Oh, um, yeah. Well I wasn't going to say." Julie responds. "I blocked his social profile from ever showing up on yours or your kid's. I wanted to see what she looked like. So Rob and I compared, and she has nothing on you."

I sighed. These two have nothing but my best interest at heart. I should probably be mad at them, but I would do the same. Maureen could look like Halle Berry or Megan Fox, but they would still say I was the more attractive one.

"Well he does work with a lot of women, and he often goes on business dinners with them." I remember him telling me that once, I think.

"Yes, I am aware of that." Julie sighs. "Business dinners do not involve holding hands, feeding each other, and quick pecks on the lips. I am so glad you are done with him."

My stomach churned. Was he doing the same thing to this new woman that he did to me? Does he even really care how he singlehandedly has changed my life? For that matter does he care anything about me at all? I had him meet my kids. How was I so stupid? Does he care he could ruin this new woman's life?

"Mandy, you still there? What's up? I know it might be hard hearing this, I wanted to make sure you realized how much of a jerk he is. You are over him, right? Mandy? Hello?"

"He gave me herpes." I blurt out.

It was dead silence on the phone. Then countdown. 5, 4, 3, 2, 1…

"THAT MOTHERFUCKING COCK SUCKING PIECE OF SHIT!"

Not sure if that was Julie, Rob, or both. It was all a blur. Between them yelling, and my thinking about other women falling prey to him. My head was buzzing.

"We are coming over there now. Rob, I will pick you up, so we are not stopped by the police. I have to make a phone call first."

Julie's call comment snaps me out of my void. "Wait, Julie, please don't do anything, he's really not worth it. Please let me tell you the whole story."

"I really CANNOT believe you are defending this asshole. Seriously! All that talk about loving you, meeting us, meeting your kids. You meeting his brother! He wanted you to stop dating other people! He gives you herpes and tosses you aside? Wait! Did he tell you he was getting married before or after he gave you herpes?"

"Hold that thought." Rob interrupts, "I think we really need to be with her now Julie. Let's stop delaying. We are on our way."

It seems as if they are teleported over, they arrive so quickly. They use the key to come in the house, and walk straight back to my room. They remove their coats to reveal pajamas, and climb on my bed. I begin my tale. Rob has a box of tissues ready. I somehow manage to tell them everything.

"I'm not understanding." Julie states. "So you can get herpes from oral sex? When NO cold sores are present? Are you fucking kidding me? Why don't more people know this?"

"Yes, it was a surprise to me, trust me. As long as I have known him, I have never seen a breakout. He also told me he doesn't remember having one, although that could very well be a lie. However the virus can shed when sores are not present. The oral one tends to shed after dental work. When I spoke to the doctor, he told me he could have it genitally, and not know it. Condoms don't protect against herpes. I don't think it was genital, or he would have infected his current girlfriend - fiancée." I correct myself. "They really don't tell you that either. HSV1 is supposed to be mild, but my vagina has felt like it was an oil fire. His doctor never tested him for it because his doctor wrongly assumed you can't pass HSV1 to others."

"And you didn't tell us this in the beginning because...." Rob asks.

"Well I thought I was going to test negative and didn't want to worry you two. When I found out I was positive was around the time your Mom was in the hospital. Me contracting herpes is not as significant as your Mom having a heart attack"

"Perhaps. But you went through this all by yourself and didn't have to, please never do this again." Rob states. "Can we make a contract. No matter what the others are going through, if we are going through something emotional we will still share?"

"Agreed." Julie states. I just manage to nod my head.

"So this asshole is possibly passing it on to someone else who doesn't know?" Rob asks. "And it affects men as well? Jesus! What about all the teenagers who think oral sex is safe? Even the gay community. That is a lot of what we do."

"I would just hate myself if someone else was going through this and I did nothing to stop it."

"I'll stop it! That fucking insensitive asshole." Julie interrupts.

"Wait, Julie, please don't have anyone disappear or anything, I just couldn't live with that either. I just would feel really guilty knowing I could've stopped someone from going through what I went through."

"Fine!" Julie sighs. "I have ways of finding out who she was, and letting her know, so she could run for the hills."

After two hours, we finally fall asleep. I cry myself to sleep as Rob holds me. The tears this time are from a better place. I realize that I am no longer alone.

Chapter 53

I wake up to Rob serving me breakfast in bed. "Hey darling! It's time to get up. We have stuff for you to do today, don't argue. I will drag you out of the bed and dress you myself."

I knew by the tone of his voice that he is serious. You never question or doubt him when he has that tone.

"It is Saturday, don't you have work today?" I ask teasingly.

"Sure do, but you're my family, you come first. I just have to call a couple of junior associates and dump my work on them."

I scoff down my eggs benedict, wanting to lick the plate. Rob only knows how to cook a handful of meals, but the ones he does cook are amazing. Plus eating diet food these pass couple of weeks, makes me appreciate the decadent dishes that come with sauces even more.

I finish eating in silence. Rob takes away the dishes, and I jump in the shower. I shower quickly, get dressed and make my way to the living room. I find Rob and Julie sitting there waiting. I would be nervous except I feel a powerful sense of love in the room.

"All ready? Let's go!"

"Wait, I have to see where my kids are." I reply.

"No need. I gave them several gift cards, and a chauffeured limousine to take them and friends around for the day. The limousine is bullet-proof, and the driver is trained in Krav Maga. He has strict instructions to protect them at all costs."

I smile. Julie could probably take over the country with her connections if she wanted to. She crosses t's and dots i's with an efficiency I have never witnessed in anyone else.

We get in Julie's car and she turns on the radio to the 70's music. Normally I would start singing with them, but I am just not in the mood. We finally pull into a parking lot.

"Listen, Amanda, we knew there was something wrong with you for a while. We couldn't figure it out. You've been going through this for a while by yourself, and you don't have to anymore. This is a support group for people with HSV. We thought it would help. We just ask that you attend a couple of meetings before you decide if you want to stay. This group wants you to come with someone each meeting. Preferably the partner that infected you, but we seriously doubt that will happen. Nor do we want him around you anymore."

I wanted to jump out the car and make a run for it. The only problem was they went through all this trouble, in a short period of time.

I let out a sigh. "Okay, let's get this over with."

Chapter 54

We walk into the building, and to a registration table. Rob handles the registration process as Julie holds my hand. We are told we are the first to arrive, and we are instructed to a classroom. We are handed different colored name tags, I guess blue for those with herpes and orange for their support.

The registration lady must have read my face. "We separate the name tags, so we know who to pay more attention to. In the past we have had some people make it all about them, when it didn't need to be. We also need you to sign this confidentiality statement. It basically says you won't divulge anyone from the group's identity."

I am about to sign the paper when Rob grabs it and ever the lawyer pursues the document. He is probably the only one I know that reads the Terms and Conditions before downloading software.

"Ok, now you may sign."

Julie and Rob of course pick seats where we can see people before they walk through the doors, but they could not see us. We often like to people watch and make up stories. Next to arrive are a group of 2 attractive and well-dressed Black women. They are holding hands, until one walks to the registration table.

"Lesbians?" I whisper.

"What is with you heteros?" Rob asks teasingly, "You see a group of same gender people and if they display any type of affection, you think they're doing each other. No, not getting the lesbian vibe from them. The one at the registration table is definitely a lawyer. Besides, how do you think WE look to people?"

"How can you tell she's a lawyer?" I ask.

"She grabbed the contract from her friend too and read it." Julie laughs.

"I've seen her before, not quite sure where." Rob answers.

"If they start fucking singing "We are the World", or "Kumbaya," I am fucking out of here." I hear one of them say. I glanced at her tag and see she has a blue one like me. I hear you sister I think.

"Just give it a try, that's all I'm asking." Her friend replies.

Ah, a kindred spirit, I bet she and I will have a lot to talk about.

"Oh, hello." The possible lawyer says "I'm Sherell, this is Ana."

As Julie introduces our group, Ana and I engage in non-verbal communication. We both tell each other we were used, and then pretty much tossed aside once we were infected. We just want to be by ourselves, but our friends are dragging us to this. We don't want to disappoint them, but still want to bolt for the door.

"Excuse me." Rob questions the possible lawyer. "You're a

lawyer aren't you?"

"Yes, I am." Sherell replies, "I was actually going to ask you the same. Were you at the ABA fundraiser in June?"

"Yes! That's where we met." Rob replies.

"Yeah, my friend tried to hit on you. I told her you were gay, but she didn't believe me." Sherell responds. "You let her down gently."

Rob smiles. "Yeah, if I cross over, I'm promised to these two." He says as he motions he head towards Julie and me.

Our group continues to talk and share stories. More people begin to arrive. Mostly in couples. A group of two men are the last to arrive, all 4 of us turn to Rob with a questioning look on our faces, and he just rolls his eyes and nods his head.

The couple at the registration table finally comes in the room. "We are ready to begin." The woman starts. "My name is Ann, and this is my husband Bob. We happen to be clinical psychologists. I however, unfortunately infected Bob with HSV1. We had a lot of stress placed on our relationship, but we worked it out, and we have never been happier. This virus is not a virus that attacks specific genders, races, or religions. You can see from the room, there is a wide variety of people. I have to implore that this a trust circle, you must respect everyone's confidentiality while you are part of the group. Any infraction and you will be asked to leave. People falsely believe you can pass on the virus, only if sores are present. Our goal is to let people know that they are not alone, and to inform the mass public of their misinformation. A million new cases occur every year, and we want to stop it before it starts. What we are going to do is go around the room and introduce ourselves and tell your story of how you got here. We also ask that you introduce the support that you have with you. We will not put you on the spot, we will ask for volunteers. We may not get to everyone the first session, but hope you continue to come back."

Everyone freezes for a good couple of seconds. I see Ana stand up with the grace and confidence of a dancer. She says, "I'll break the ice. I guess you just want a summary and not the specific details. Or we'll be here all day?"

"We and your loved ones are here, as long as you need us to be. A summary is fine, the specific details will come out later."

She tells a story similar to mine. She was with a guy who was seeing someone else. She said he never had a cold sore. She wasn't too worried going through the testing, as she saw a Dr. Oz show on cold sores, and he stated they are transmitted by spores that are present when the sores are present on the lip. So she was shocked when she received the bad news. Ditto I think to myself.

At one point she started crying, and had to sit down. Her friend immediately grabbed her hand for support. She goes on to say she actually enjoyed sex. Even masturbation, and now she cannot even think about it. She explains how she went through this by herself, the guy even ditched a discussion they were going to have to go see movie. She goes on to say he finally delivered the hatchet via instant messenger.

I look at the other couples that were there. They seem to look lovingly and appreciatively in each other's eyes. They must be here with the person that infected them. I realized that once Ana was done, I had to go next, or I would never be able to go after the lovey-dovey couples.

Once she was done, she collapsed into the arms of her friend.

"Thank you Ana, for your story. You were very brave to go first."

"Who would like to go next?"

I volunteer and go through my nightmare. It was somewhat easier for me, as I had just shared the story with Julie and Rob the night before. I could see the sympathetic looks from the others in the room. It was quite annoying actually. I zeroed in on Ana. She got me. There was no sympathetic look on face. More like a "If you need me to slash some tires, I'm there for you." I gave her a "back at you smile." And she smiled letting me know we understood each other. I even threw in being supportive of Michael when he thought his girlfriend had HPV. I gave Julie and Rob a "sorry forgot to tell you look."

Once I was done, the gentleman from the "gay" male couple stood up. Rick was there with his brother Sam. We all looked at Rob, and he just shrugged his shoulders. He was infected by a female partner - a Pentecostal. After his running around, and finally finding information on the web, he said he was willing to work things out, but she blamed everything on Satan, and did not want to listen. I see Ana and Sherell roll their eyes. I guess her group was not a religious one.

Once Rick was finished, one more couple went for the day. It was another man, but he was there with his wife. They were both shocked and disturbed when they heard the news. They immediately suspected the other of cheating. But after marriage counseling and internet research, they realized there was no infidelity in the marriage. There was only a few minutes left, so the wife had a chance to speak. She spoke of her guilt of passing it on, and how she would apologize to him every day. She then said she realized that was getting annoying, so she would go out of her way to show how much she really cared for him and how sorry she was. She would make appointments for doctors, and she found the support group.

After the meeting, Ana's, Rick's and my group mingled. We talked about how we were tired of crying, and the guilt of crying, as there were people with worse ailments. Ana admitted she would have a hard time dating again. She just didn't want to open herself up to anyone like that again. Rick agreed and mentioned not wanting to have to explain this to someone – as if they would believe HSV1 was not so bad, and lots of people have it and test positive for it. I admitted that I would have difficulty trusting someone again.

We all agreed that it drove us crazy that doctors had a nonchalant attitude about it, and how more people are not aware. Oral sex is the "choice du jour" for a lot of young people, and even people who meet for quick flings. Because unfortunately "oral sex really sex isn't sex." We all rolled our eyes and sighed.

We finally had to part ways, but the entire group agreed to exchange emails in case anyone needed to vent until we met again. Or came across any information we wanted to share. Such as that new gynecologist I have yet to find.

"Soooooooo?" Asked Rob. "Michael's girlfriend had HPV?"

"No she tested negative." I respond.

"Yes, but during your story you mentioned the doctor said sometimes they confuse the two." Rob replies.

"Yes but she tested…." Wait I think to myself as I notice Rob and Julie nodding heads, that bastard probably knew all along he had HSV1.

I see Julie about to say something and I interrupt her. "No Julie, I do not want him to disappear. I do not want to break them up. Yes he is an asshole, but she doesn't seem to think so. Why mess with her fantasy?"

I see she is about to say something else, so I interrupt her again, silently giggling to myself. NO ONE interrupts her. If I never knew before how much she loved me, I know now.

237

"Well I enjoyed the group, meeting Ana and Rick. They're so young. It's a shame that this could've been prevented. It worries me that no one knows about this."

"Hey! If they have a vaccine for chicken pox, why don't they have a vaccine/cure for herpes." Rob asks. "I mean the virus is similar right?"

"Welllllllll, there is a cure in the works." Julie states.

"What?!" I gasp. "You were going to share this when?"

"Well that is the bad part. There is a researcher, a Dr. Cullen at Duke University who has found a possible cure, but he needs funding. A million dollars. More would also help."

"WOW!" Rob responds. "That is nothing in the pharmaceutical world. Talk about your pharmaceutical conspiracy. I'd be all over that if I owned a company. But they make more money curing flare-ups than they do the actually disease."

My mind begins to race. How to raise money and make people aware. I whip out my blackberry and begin to plug in everyone's email from the support group. I then send them all an email asking if they would be willing to share their story for a book. The book can be used as a fundraiser for Dr. Cullen's research and as well as a warning to others.

Ana is the first to respond. "I actually have all the text messages/IM chats/emails and blood test results saved."

I smile. A true woman. We tend to save all that crap don't we?

Rick responds next. "That sounds like a good place to start. I'd be more than happy to participate. Perhaps I can work on a webpage, and a facebook page?"

I begin to receive more emails from the rest of the group. One has even found an awareness ribbon.

"Who are you texting?" Rob asks.

"The group. We're writing a book. There is currently no book that talks about preventing herpes or about a cure. We're doing it. All it takes is one. This time one group." I respond.

BZZZZZZZ. My cell phone buzzing briefly stopped the conversation. I saw it was a text message from John.

"Amanda babes! I talked to Michael. He told me he was getting married. Asshole! I can't believe it, as much crap as he talks about her. The guys are done with him. Next game there is no mention of him. EVER. We all apologize, he had us fooled."

I smile. It was nice to hear his apology and know that although the guys did not know the entire story, they were on my side.

"That's a good idea." Julie beams. "A book. "A book would be more global. I'm sure this just isn't happening in the US. People need to know so they can protect themselves properly and make wise decisions. What can we do to help?"

"Well, right now, just have my back, which I know I don't have to ask for as you two always do and I love you for it. Ana and Rick agreed to meet at my house tomorrow, so we can start an outline."

And just like that, Amanda Jones was born.

Chapter 55

We now ask that you do a web search – to see the other people scratching their heads wondering how this happened to them. You'll see posts from all around the world. Then decide for yourself when a doctor tells you there is a slim chance of this happening to you. It doesn't matter which search engine you use, you'll see the stories.

Things you should know about herpes and actions you should take to prevent contracting it:

1. You cannot contact the virus from a toilet seat, or sharing towels.
2. If you are in a relationship, you are your partner should get tested IMMEDIATELY. If one of you tests positive for HSV1, have the talk and decide if oral sex is an option for you two. *Remember, one of the authors was infected by someone who never had a cold sore.*
3. You are not safe from HSV1 or HSV2 using condoms. Condoms move. You are also not safe just because there are no sores present. The virus can be passed by something called "shedding." There are medications you can take to

help limit the transmission, but again this is another topic of conversation if you or your partner is infected.

4. If you are just new to a relationship. Go get tested together. Look at each other's results. Make it a date if need be. If your partner does not want to go, get rid of them. Chances are they are hiding something. You must ASK to be tested for HSV1 and HSV2. Many places do not do it automatically. A complete STD test should include: Chlamydia, Gonorrhea, HIV, HPV, HSV1, HSV2, Hepatitis, Syphilis, Genital Warts, Vaginitis. Many places do not test for crabs or pubic lice, because that is something you can usually see on your own.

5. This is a tricky one. If you test positive for HSV1, you are immune from contracting HSV1. If you test positive for HSV2, you are immune from contracting HSV2. However, if you have HSV1, you can still contract HSV2, and if you have HSV2, you can still contract HSV1.

6. This is even trickier. If you have HSV1 genital, you can pass it on to someone who does not carry the virus by having sexual intercourse. You can pass HSV1 from genital to genital, or mouth to genital.

7. Stop wasting money on the natural cures you see on line. Instead invest your money in legitimate research. Visit http://www.oralstd.webs.com/ for information on research.

8. Write your local politicians and ask why are HSV1 and HSV2 not considered medical conditions, where recent studies have shown links to Alzheimer's disease. Pregnant women can have miscarriages because of the virus. Acne medications are covered. Why not HSV?

9. If you are in a country outside of the USA, and we hope this book travels the world, so everyone becomes more aware, put the pressure on your department or ministers of health. Demand answers. We have been in the dark long enough.

10. If someone you are in a relationship tells you they have herpes, don't have a meltdown on them. Be thankful that

they told you so you will have options that they perhaps did not.

ABOUT THE AUTHOR

Insert author bio text here. Insert author bio text here